Making Health Care Whole

Making Health Care Whole

Integrating Spirituality into Health Care

Christina M. Puchalski, MD

Betty Ferrell, RN, PhD

FOREWORD BY
RACHEL NAOMI REMEN, MD

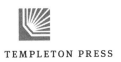

TEMPLETON PRESS

Templeton Press

300 Conshohocken State Road, Suite 550

West Conshohocken, PA 19428

www.templetonpress.org

Library of Congress Cataloging-in-Publication Data
Puchalski, Christina M.
Making health care whole : integrating spirituality into health
care / Christina M. Puchalski, Betty Ferrell.
p. ; cm.
Includes bibliographical references and index.
ISBN-13: 978-1-59947-350-5 (pbk. : alk. paper)
ISBN-10: 1-59947-350-X (pbk. : alk. paper)   1. Palliative
treatment.   2. Spirituality.   3. Spiritual healing.   4. Medicine—
Religious aspects.   I. Ferrell, Betty.   II. Title.
[DNLM: 1. Palliative Care—standards—Guideline.
2. Professional Role—Guideline.   3. Religion and Medicine—
Guideline.   4. Spirituality—Guideline. WB 310 P977m 2010]
R726.8.P83 2010
616´.029—dc22
2009046709

Designed and typeset by Kachergis Book Design

Printed in the United States of America

10   11   12   13   14   15   10   9   8   7   6   5   4   3   2   1

The authors dedicate this book to Rose Mary Carroll Johnson, MN, RN. Her expert skill as an editor came to us at a pivotal time and her gifts helped us to make our consensus conference and this book a reality.

The authors also acknowledge the contribution of content by our key advisors:

Harvey Chochinov, MD, PhD, FRCPC

Holly Nelson-Becker, PhD, MSW

Karen Pugliese, MA, BCC

George Handzo, MDiv, MA, BCC

Maryjo Prince-Paul, PhD, APRN, AHPCN

Daniel Sulmasy, OFM, MD, PhD

Contents

Figures

Tables

Foreword

Rachel Naomi Remen, MD

As health professionals our relationship with the spiritual dimension of life is intimate but often unaware. This became clear to me some years ago when I was a part of a seminar Joseph Campbell ran for physicians on the experience of spiritual reality. The doctors who had gathered together were uncomfortable with the topic, uncertain of what spiritual reality had to do with us and with our work. Recognizing this, Campbell opened the session by projecting images of sacred art on a screen before us, paintings and sculpture and tapestries.

One of these works remains clear in my memory, a small bronze of a dancing Shiva, the god of creation, from a museum in Europe. I remember being struck by the beauty and joy of the little figure, dancing with abandon in a ring of bronze flame, one foot lifted high in the air and the other resting on the back of a little man, crouched in the dust, completely absorbed in something that he was holding between his hands. Looking more closely, I could see that the focus of his attention was a leaf. Others, too, were struck by the beauty of the figure, but we were all trained observers and posers of questions and so one of us spoke up and asked Campbell, "What is that little man doing there?"

"Aha," Campbell exclaimed, "That little man is someone who is so caught up in the study of the material world that he does not know that the living god is dancing on his back."

There was a long silence and Campbell looked at us sitting there in our white coats, suits and ties . . . and smiled.

There is little in our highly technological training that encourages us to recognize or respond to spiritual reality, yet the spirit is a part of our daily lives as health professionals. Our medical culture often limits the ways that we think, the ways that we see things. It interprets our experience for us in ways that are often constricted and small. But life is larger than these interpretations, more filled with mystery and wonder and awe. More worthy of gratitude. Things happen that cannot be predicted or measured or even explained, things that cannot be controlled but only witnessed. When we become fully present at such times, we open a doorway of meaning and possibility for our patients and for ourselves as well.

In essence, we have traded mystery for mastery and paid a great price. We have lost the ability to meet honestly with the unknown to wonder together with our patients on the deeper meanings of things, to share questions as well as answers. We have forgotten how to listen.

Mystery is not an idea, it is an experience—a willingness to let the mask of habit that makes things familiar fall away in order to catch a glimpse of something different. The head of a large urban emergency room once told me of such an epiphany in his work. It had been a busy night on his service and he was called to attend to a woman about to deliver a baby. A quick examination confirmed that the delivery was so imminent that there was no time to call an obstetrician, no time to even move her from the gurney into a treatment room. So with nurses holding her legs on their shoulders he successfully delivered her little girl right there in the ambulance bay of the emergency room.

"Rachel," he told me, "this was the sort of thing I used to pride myself on, intense experiences that confirmed me in my sense of myself, my skill, and my technique."

"And this was different?" I asked him.

"Very." he replied.

The delivery had gone perfectly. He was holding the baby below the placenta with the back of her head in his palm, suctioning her nose and mouth, when suddenly the infant's eyes opened and she looked deeply into his eyes. In that moment he stepped past his usual way of seeing and realized a simple thing: he was the first human being that this tiny child had ever seen. He felt his heart go out to her in welcome and was surprised to discover tears in his eyes. In that moment years of cynicism, numbness, and resentment simply vanished and were replaced by an unfamiliar feeling. It took him two days to identify it but eventually he recognized that it was gratitude for being the person who got to welcome her.

We both fell silent. "A holy moment, Rachel," he told me. "I've missed a lot of them. So I look for them on purpose now and they are everywhere."

As health professionals we often meet people at the thresholds of the world, welcoming them when they are born and letting go of their hands as they die. Yet little in our training prepares us to have comfort with the unknown or even to recognize the spiritual nature of such meetings. Many of us still question whether "spirit" is an appropriate concern of health professionals, daunted by the word itself with its whiff of holiness, its sense of being the prerogative of those who are expert in such matters, specially trained or even called. But what if "spirit" is seen in another way, as a dimension in all relationships and all people, a yearning for a larger connection and a deeper meaning that is just a natural part of our being? What if we could learn to trust a part of ourselves that is not acquired but inborn, unashamed by a lack of explainability? What if we could let go of the need to understand and simply be there for one another?

Years ago a man with terminal cancer who came to one of Commonweal's cancer retreats pressed a poem into my hand as he left. He had crafted it from the words of others because it spoke of his experience of mystery and healing at the end of life and the relationship he hoped to find with the professionals who accompanied him there and cared for him.

> I had a dream
> That honeybees were making honey in my heart,
> out of my old failures.
> There is no wrong or right.
> Beyond the wrong and the right, there is a field.
> I'll meet you there.

Embracing the mystery in our work may require us to first heal the wounds of our training. The way I was trained, the father of health care could easily have been John Wayne. Reality was narrowly defined and for many years I believed that anything real was evidence based, and what could be described in numbers was truer than what could only be described in words. But perhaps the things that are most real are those that cannot be expressed in numbers or even words but only directly known. Our lives are transformed by such experiences.

Sometimes life-threatening illness may be the setting in which such a transformative experience of may occur.

In the process of treatment for recurrent cancer, one of my patients underwent a radical transformation. As a child of atheistic and intellectual parents, he had no religious upbringing or spiritual inclination and had immersed himself in the world of competition and business with much success. While formerly his business had been the focus of his life, now his cancer and its treatment required him to spend several months in the quiet of his living room.

As the fatigue of his chemotherapy took hold, he simply surrendered to this silence and spent hours on his couch dozing in the company of his cat. One afternoon, as he lay drifting in and out of sleep, he found himself looking at the opposite wall and it seemed to him that one of the books on the bookshelf stood out from the others in an odd way. Getting up for a closer look he saw that it was the Bible that the clergy who had performed his marriage years ago had given to him and his wife. Taking it back to the couch he opened it for the first time and started to read the story of the beginning of the world. He was surprised to feel a deep response to the simple words, how real and familiar and terrifying the formlessness and darkness felt to him and how it seemed to be somehow connected to the recent events in his life. And then he encountered the statement with which the world begins: "*Let there be light.*" He lay there for a time feeling the great power in these words wash over him.

As he ruminated about this, he suddenly realized that these words were addressed to him personally, that he could act in ways that increased the light in the world. He had never considered this possibility before but over the next days and weeks it became a more and more compelling thought, until he recognized it as a deep yearning in himself to live in a certain way. That perhaps the goal of life was not to be wealthy or succeed in business or to leave a financial inheritance to his children as he had thought. Perhaps he might use whatever time was left to him to bring more light into the world. Perhaps this was the inheritance he could leave to his children.

Life-threatening illness may encourage a return to that which is most genuine in each of us. It may initiate a turning away from a false self, the person whom we have been taught to be or whom others have wanted us to be, to embrace the person we most deeply are for the first time. As such, the end of life may be a healing, a movement toward an integrity that is unique for each one of us. At times of significant illness a door may open and the familiar may fall away to be replaced by something never before seen but always known and deeply recognized. These doors open only one way. Once this is seen there is no going back. These transformations are often spiritual in nature. In such moments of profound change it is as if our true life is offered to us, a life transparent to our deepest values.

Working with such people at the edge of life may change our sense of perspective and task. It may cause us to see health care as a spiritual path and ourselves as spiritual beings. A colleague, a prominent cancer surgeon in our community, made this discovery in a dramatic way through his own experience of life-threatening illness. Some years ago he was shocked to discover that he had a malignancy and needed cancer surgery. He had never been ill before and he took this as a personal affront. Unwilling to reveal his vulnerability to his colleagues and students he took a vacation, arranged to be hospitalized at another institution, and persuaded his wife to tell no one.

A few months after this surgery, he stopped by my office in response to an invitation to lunch. I commented that he seemed different to me and he shared his recent experience and how it had changed the way in which he saw himself and his work. He told me that when he had awakened in the recovery room, he was in such severe pain that he was astounded. As he lay there overwhelmed by pain he slowly became aware of another experience, a sense of peace so profound that it felt more like a sort of trust.

"Trust of what, Harold?" I asked him.

He fell silent. "I guess a trust of life itself," he told me.

Comforted he had let himself surrender into this peace, all the while experiencing the most horrific pain. And then a phrase from his childhood came back to him—"The peace that surpasseth all understanding"—and he found himself wondering if this was an experience of that peace. Certain that it was, he was filled with a profound gratitude for having found in himself the capacity to experience it.

"How extraordinary," I told him.

"Yes," he said, but this was only the beginning. Lying there, he had recognized becoming the most skillful surgeon and the most admired physician in his community was not his real work. His real work was simply cultivating in himself this sense of deep peace and trust of life, bringing it with him into places of fear and suffering, holding it in himself so steady that others might be able to feel it in him, to trust it and take refuge in it in dark times just as he was taking refuge in it now.

Perhaps our best work as health professionals is not about something we do but about something we are, something we become and bring into all our relationships. Perhaps others can recognize what we bring to them because it is the direction in which they are already moving. Perhaps in our presence they can move in that direction less afraid.

Entering the spiritual realm with someone at the end of life often does not require special expertise or training; it may simply require us to listen without judgment and to ask a few of the simplest of questions. Rather than seeking ways to introduce the concept of spirit to people at such times, we may simply need to remember that we and our patients are already on spiritual ground and become willing to listen and to wonder together. Questions of a spiritual nature often arise spontaneously at the close of a lifetime. "What matters now?" "What is really important?" "What can be trusted"? Simply asking such questions aloud may become an invitation to shared discovery and a deeper connection. People often have spontaneous thoughts or dreams or memories of spiritual importance that they are willing to share as well.

One of my patients, an internationally known architect, shared such a memory with his wife and me late one afternoon as we sat on either side of his hospital bed in the little study of his home. At the time he was desperately sick with cancer and waiting to find out if his latest tests would show that there was further treatment available for him. It did not seem likely. The house was still and as we sat together I could feel the weight of his wife's anxiety and his own as well. I felt a longing for a place of ease and safety, just a few moments of respite. I imagine that we all did.

As he lay in bed, struggling to breathe, I asked him if he could remember a place or time when he had felt safe. Without hesitation, he began to describe his childhood, the fields and the woods, the sound of the birds at sunrise, and then he remembered a story. It had happened when he was very small and lived in a house at the end of a dirt road that ran alongside a small river.

Often in spring the river would flood. Once as he was walking along the road after a flood he found a rainbow trout, washed up from the river, struggling to live in the shallow drainage ditch. Small as he was, he was horrified by this beautiful fish, trapped and struggling in too small a place. It was a big fish but somehow he managed to get it up into his arms. Carrying it across the road, he waded into the river a little ways and set it free. Deeply moved, I asked him what he remembered most clearly about this. He said he remembered the moment when the fish between his hands realized it was once again part of the river.

There are many meanings in every story. On one level this is a beautiful childhood memory shared by a very sick man. On another it is a story about a man whose compassion goes back to his very beginnings. But I think there may be deeper readings still.

Certain practices run through all the branches of Buddhism. One of these celebrates the promise of enlightenment and freedom from suffering. In China, Japan, Nepal, and Korea, live fish are bought at the market, taken to bodies of running water, and set free. These fish symbolize the promise of a return to the Source that is our true home.

There is also a Buddhist teaching concerning the death of one who has accumulated the power to free others and help them to live well. The death of such a one is called "taking on the Rainbow Body" and it is believed that at death the physical bodies of such men and women vanish into a rainbow of light.

This man was not a Buddhist. He did not know any of this intellectually. He was an architect, a vintner, a fly fisherman, a sailor, a friend, a husband, and a father. But there was in him, as there is in us all, something that went deeper than all these things, an unconscious wisdom that was very old. "If we are quiet and listen, sometimes, without our knowing, it speaks to us directly."

And so, as we were waiting together, anxious and fearful, hoping to find that further treatment was available, I think that this part in him told all three of us this story. Perhaps it spoke to us so that we would know where he was in his life or, even more important, so that we would understand that despite appearances, all was well.

Over many years of listening to terminally ill people, their dreams, their poems, their stories, I have come across many images for the soul, some conscious and many unconscious. I think the rainbow trout is one of the most beautiful.

Perhaps the care of the dying is not about the care of the body but the care of the soul. This presents a bit of a quandary to those trained in the skills of physical medicine. It may leave us shifting from foot to foot, anxious and uncertain for the task ahead, and cause us to fall back on treatments and medications that are both inappropriate and unwise. Little in our training encourages us to accept the limitations of our science and trust the power of relationships that are simply human, or to be at peace with things that we cannot understand, or to have the patience to wait for a natural unfolding and revelation. We are trained to fix and control, to anticipate and analyze. But the dying are not broken and everything we cannot understand may not be awry.

Caring for the soul requires that we be fully present in situations we cannot control and patient as a genuine meaning and a direction unfold. It means seeing familiar things in new ways, listening rather than speaking, learning from patients rather than teaching them, and cultivating the capacity to be amazed. It means recognizing the power of our own humanity to make a difference in the lives of others and valuing it as highly as our expertise. Finally, it means discovering that health care is a front-row seat on mystery and sitting in that seat with open eyes.

Making Health Care Whole is a gift to all health care professionals who yearn to go beyond the limitations of their training and practice their work as a calling. It enables us to be open to the mystery in our work and offers us a practical model and the tools to serve the unmet needs of our patients. It offers us permission to tend to our own souls and to grow in wisdom as well as in knowledge through this work. It can make us as well as our medicine more whole.

Preface

During the past fifteen years, there has been growing interest in and attention to spiritual care as a dimension of palliative care services. This book is based on a consensus conference and associated project activities built on nationally peer-reviewed guidelines that were developed by the National Consensus Project for Quality Palliative Care (NCP, 2004) and endorsed by key national palliative care organizations to provide spiritual care for seriously ill and dying patients. While the NCP guidelines recognize spirituality as an essential dimension of palliative care, uniformity of spiritual care practice is lacking across health care settings. Barriers to standardized implementation include varying understandings and definitions of spirituality, lack of resources and practical tools, and limited professional education and training in spiritual care.

The purpose of the consensus conference was to establish a common language and model for interdisciplinary spiritual care, identify resources and tools that have practical applications for health care settings, and develop recommendations that will advance the practice of spiritual care in palliative care settings. Achieving a consensus on spiritual care, both conceptually and pragmatically, requires engagement, deliberation, and dialogue among key stakeholders. Conference participation was by invitation. Invitees included a representative sample of forty national leaders, encompassing physicians, nurses, psychologists, social workers, chaplains and clergy, other spiritual care providers, and health care administrators. Over the following months, a consensus document was revised yet again to incorporate the feedback from conference participants. The version of the document was sent to a panel of 150 expert reviewers for additional comments.

While the focus of the conference was on palliative care, because palliative care is defined from the time someone is diagnosed with a serious illness, the material in this book is applicable to most care across the life cycle. Support for this consensus document and consensus conference has been provided by the Archstone Foundation, a private grant-making organization whose mission is to prepare society for an aging population. The goal of this document is to advance the practice of spiritual care and inform future policy and research efforts.

1 INTRODUCTION AND OVERVIEW

Part 1 sets forth the background, research,
historical, ethical, and philosophical contexts
and organizational standards in place that
support the importance of spirituality in
palliative care and health care in general.

1 Why Spirituality in Palliative Care

I realized that we needed not only better pain control but better overall care. People needed the space to be themselves. I coined the term "total pain," from my understanding that dying people have physical, spiritual, psychological, and social pain that must be treated. I have been working on that ever since.

Cecily Saunders, MD (as quoted in Smith, 2005)

Cecily Saunders, the founder of hospice and palliative care, speaks to the core of what spirituality means in the care of all patients, particularly those suffering from chronic illness and facing their own death. People deserve "total care" where they can speak authentically about their illness and where their spiritual needs as well as their physical, social, and emotional needs are addressed. Illness, aging, and the prospect of dying can trigger profound questions about who people are, what their life has meant, and what will become of them during the course of their illness and perhaps after they die. Who am I? How will I be remembered? These questions have the same importance in patients' lives as do questions about treatment. Illness and dying are essentially spiritual processes in that they often provoke deep questions of meaning, purpose, and hope. These questions can trigger a quest for answers. That quest is what many would call a spiritual journey and why some consider palliative care to be a "secular religious movement" (Duffy, 2009).

Viktor Frankl wrote that "man is not destroyed by suffering; he is destroyed by suffering without meaning" (Frankl, 1963). Spirituality helps give meaning to suffering and helps people find hope in the midst of despair. In the midst of suffering, a skillful, caring, and compassionate health care professional can be an important anchor in which the patient can find solace and the strength to move through distress to peace and acceptance.

Studies of Spirituality and Health Outcomes in Palliative Care

Research in palliative care has demonstrated the impact of religious and spiritual beliefs on people's moral decision making, way of life, interactions with others, life choices, and ability to transcend suffering and to deal with life's challenges. Spirituality is broadly defined as that which gives meaning and purpose to life and is often a central issue for patients at the end of life or those dealing with chronic illness (Puchalski et al., 2004; Astrow et al., 2001; King et al., 1994). Every individual makes decisions as to whether life has meaning and value that extends beyond self, life, and death. Dealing with these existential questions focuses on a relationship with a transcendent being or concept (Sulmasy, 1999). Spirituality and religious beliefs have been shown to have an impact on how people cope with serious illness and life stresses. Spiritual practices can foster coping resources (Koenig et al., 2001; Roberts et al., 1997), promote health-related behavior (Powell et al., 2003), enhance a sense of well-being and improve quality of life (Cohen et al., 1996), provide social support (Burgener, 1999), and generate feelings of love and forgiveness (Worthington, 2001). Spiritual beliefs can also affect health care decision making (Silvestri et al., 2003). However, spiritual/religious beliefs can also create distress and increase the burdens of illness (Koenig et al., 1998).

The notion that spirituality is central to the dying person is well recognized by many experts, the most important being those patients who are seriously ill. A 1997 Gallup survey of a random sample of American religious and nonreligious adults showed that people overwhelmingly want to reclaim and reassert the spiritual dimensions when dying. Survey respondents said they wanted warm relationships with their health care providers, to be listened to, to have someone to share fears and concerns with, to have someone with them when they are dying, to be able to pray and have others pray for them, and to have a chance to say good-bye to loved ones. When asked what would worry them, respondents said not being forgiven by God or others, or having continued emotional and spiritual suffering. When asked what would bring them comfort, they reported wanting to believe that death is a normal part of the life cycle and that they would live on through their relationships, accomplishments, or good works. They also wanted to believe that they had done their best in life and that they would be in the presence of a loving God or Higher Power.

It is as important for health care professionals to talk with patients about these issues as it is to address the physical aspects of care. Numerous surveys have shown patients want their caregivers to talk with them about their spiritual needs. In these surveys, 65 to 70 percent of people polled say they want their physicians to address their spiritual issues, yet only about 10 percent report actually having these conversations with their physicians (Ehman et al., 1999; McCord et al., 2004).

Surveys have also indicated that people turn to spiritual or religious beliefs in times of stress and difficulty. Particularly when people are faced with a life-threatening illness, questions about meaning and purpose in the midst of suffering arise. It is not uncommon for people to question God, fairness, and life choices. People often undertake a life review, where issues related to their life, relationships, and self-worth might arise. Spiritual issues include hopelessness, despair, guilt, shame, anger, and abandonment by God or others. These issues can provoke deep suffering, which can result from people feeling alienated from themselves, others, God, or from their ultimate source of meaning.

Suffering

Patients confronted with mortality, limitations, and loss wrestle with questions about life's purpose and meaning amidst suffering. But what is suffering? Cassell (1991) defined suffering as the state of distress brought about by an actual or perceived threat to the integrity or continued existence of the whole person. Suffering is "an anguish that is experienced, not only as a pressure to change, but as a threat to our composure, our integrity, and the fulfillment of our intentions" (Cassell, 1991, p. 231). A central notion in this definition is that those who suffer submit (or are forced to submit) to a particular set of circumstances outside of their control. Such a situation has the potential to seriously erode one's autonomy, and foster hopelessness and loss of control.

Thus, spiritual suffering may be manifested as inner distress, grief/

loss, hopelessness, worry, and isolation (Ferrell & Coyle, 2008). Wright (2005) described several experiences of suffering, including the alteration of one's life and relationships with serious illness; the forced exclusion from everyday life; the strain of trying to endure; the longing to love or be loved; enduring acute or chronic pain; and experiencing conflict, anguish, or interference with love in relationships.

Spiritual suffering may also be manifested as physical pain, depression or anxiety, social isolation, and spiritual or existential distress. Pain is multidimensional and may be exacerbated or relieved by attention to the other dimensions of suffering. Spiritual suffering or pain may manifest within various domains of the patient's experience, be it physical (e.g., intractable pain), psychological (e.g., anxiety, depression, hopelessness), religious (e.g., crisis of faith, anger at God), or social (e.g., disintegration of human relationships). Figure 1 demonstrates how patients may have varying patterns of suffering. One patient's suffering may be predominantly spiritual; another's may be mostly psychological.

Suffering is difficult to diagnose based on symptoms alone. For example, spiritual pain is the combination of these aforementioned symptoms and characteristic behaviors, including patients who are desperate to escape their situation, patients with expectations of caregivers that are impossible to meet, patients who continue to try new therapies in the absence of any benefit, and patients who require escalating doses of analgesics and sedatives despite no apparent benefit even when these measures are clearly counterproductive. These behaviors often evoke descriptions such as "suffering" or "anguish," which can signal the need for psychosocial and/or spiritual intervention (McGrath, 2002).

Some studies suggest that existential and spiritual issues may be of greater concern to patients than pain and physical symptoms (Breitbart et al., 1996; Field & Cassel, 1997). Thus, a patient's report of pain may be referring to pain in any of these dimensions. Unless the health care practitioner is attentive to all the dimensions of suffering—the psychosocial and spiritual, as well as the physical—the entire focus of care may be on physical pain while neglecting the spiritual or existential distress.

Frank was a sixty-eight-year-old male dying of pancreatic can-

FIGURE 1   Profile of Suffering

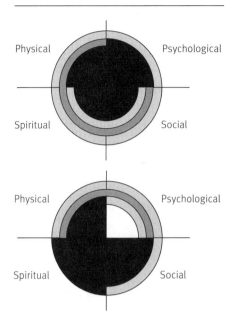

cer. He was in excruciating pain and receiving high doses of opioids, sedatives, and other pain medications. Despite the medication he continued to cry out in pain, rating his pain a "100" on a scale of 1–10. Eventually, the nursing staff became uncomfortable with the high dose of medications given and the continued pain complaints. I (Puchalski) went into his room, meeting him for the first time and asked about his life. He was reticent to tell me any personal details. I asked him if he had any spiritual resources that might help him. He readily answered that he was an Episcopalian but then got quiet and said he needed more pain medication. I was on duty for the whole week in the hospice, so I decided to again pursue this question the next day when I saw him. This time he told me he stopped going to church a long time ago for a "personal reason." I shared this information in the interdisciplinary team rounds and asked the chaplain to also work on this issue with Frank. Over the next few weeks, Frank revealed to the chaplain that he had left the church because he was a homosexual and thought they would disapprove of him. He felt isolated for many years, and now that he was dying, he thought God would not be there for him. The chaplain shared this information with the medical team and suggested ways each of us could work with Frank on the spiritual issues of guilt and the need for reconciliation and reconnection with his faith community. The chaplain worked with Frank, as did the rest of us on the team, being present to him, affirming him, and letting him know he was loved. Eventually, Frank was able to see a priest, receive the sacraments, and feel a sense of acceptance by the church community. He no longer needed huge doses of pain medication. Several months later he died in peace.

Among patients with life-threatening illness, sensing oneself as a burden to others seems to be an important theme related to quality of life, optimal palliative care, and maintenance of dignity at the end of life (Cohen & Leis, 2002; Cousineau et al., 2003; Weisman, 1972). Personal or individual autonomy—especially in Western society—is often conflated with the notion of being a whole person, so that dependency can be seen or experienced as threatening the integrity of personhood itself. Suffering can threaten the intactness of the person (Cassell, 1982). Thus, it is important to address spiritual concerns of making meaning in illness and finding a sense of dignity and purpose to help others overcome that sense of burden to others.

Spiritual Transformation in the Midst of Suffering

There are many stories and considerable anecdotal evidence indicating that some patients are able to understand their illness as an opportunity for growth and to see their life and their relationships in a way that enables them to find enhanced meaning in life that is more profound and gratifying than life prior to their illness (Puchalski, 2004). Tsevat et al. (1999) conducted focus groups with patients with HIV/AIDS and reported that many found their lives were better than before their diagnosis. Tsevat also found that most patients with HIV/AIDS were at peace with God and the universe. These researchers (Cotton et al., 2006) also demonstrated that the majority of patients with HIV/AIDS reported that spirituality is an important factor in their lives, as most indicated some sense of meaning/purpose in their lives and reported deriving comfort from their spiritual beliefs. The majority of our patients with HIV/AIDS belonged to an organized religion but participated more often in nonorganized religious activities (e.g., prayer, meditation). Similarly, patients with advanced cancer who derived comfort from their religious and spiritual beliefs were more satisfied with their lives, were happier, and reported less pain (Yates et al., 1981). Women with breast cancer said that their spiritual beliefs helped them cope with their illness and with facing death and that they "became more spiritual" as a result of their illness, reflecting a transformative process (Roberts et al., 1997).

Health care professionals also write of the transformation they experience as a result of interactions with their patients. By experiencing personal suffering, professionals may be better able to relate to and be compassionate with patients. Bolen (1996), a psychiatrist who works with individuals with severe chronic and terminal illnesses, uses the phrase "expansion of the soul" to describe the transformation that enables an empathic and compassionate connection to the suffering. Albert Schweitzer (1931) wrote of a similar transformation after he developed a serious illness. He described the profound change that he experienced spiritually after he confronted his possible death from the illness. He recognized that those who have experienced suffering may be changed spiritually, and part of the change is being awakened to a sense of duty to help others overcome their suffering. Thus, suffering becomes the trigger for spiritual transformation for the patients, and often for the clinician, which then can lead to compassion for self and for others who suffer. In our research at the City of Hope in the area of family caregivers, we have often heard stories from family members who find great meaning amidst their suffering. A father of a young boy dying of cancer said that "if this weren't the worst experience of my life, it would be the best." The father described how having a child with serious illness was a parent's worst nightmare, yet through this experience he and his wife had experienced a great strengthening of their faith, love for each other, appreciation of their church and community, and an altered view of what was truly important in life.

Caregivers can also be transformed by the suffering of loved ones or patients. When my (Puchalski) fiancé, Eric, was diagnosed with cancer, I remember thinking that my life would never be the same. It was only years later that I recognized how true that perception was, that in many ways, the suffering I witnessed and experienced myself triggered personal and spiritual changes within me that enabled me to become a better physician. Like the father of the young boy above, I experienced a deepening of my faith. I also experienced a greater commitment to my vocation as a physician and an overwhelming sense of the beauty of humanity, life, and God. I no longer feared suffering but recognized it as a natural part of life and an opportunity for growth and transition. I became passionate in my desire to support others in the midst of their suffering. Service became the foundation for my work, rather than fixing or solving others' problems; for with suffering there are no quick fixes, just patient love and partnership while the suffering patient finds the answers amidst the suffering and anger as well as joy and transformation.

Medical and nursing professionals have written about their obligation to relieve suffering. Many religious leaders and practitioners from other spiritual disciplines write of suffering as a spiritual process. While it may be possible to relieve physical suffering with medication, is the relief of spiritual suffering possible or even desirable? Perhaps spiritual care calls us to bear witness to and accompany people in their suffering and provide support as patients find meaning in the midst of that suffering and eventually integrate the suffering into their lives and become transformed by it.

Patients' search for meaning and authenticity may also affect how they comply with pain regiments. There are many anecdotal stories of patients who will choose to be in physical pain to be alert enough to spend time with their families or to be awake enough to finish the book they are writing or the poems they are creating for their children. Thus, people will place those things they hold sacred—family, God, dreams, projects—above their physical needs and even the need for pain relief. This challenges our paradigms of good quality of life and living with dying and death. Good quality care occurs when patients are able to express what is holy to them, gives them meaning, and helps them transcend their suffering, even if not necessarily relieving it (Balducci, 2008). Thus, the clinician's role becomes one of a partner or companion on the journey, rather than fixer or alleviator. One of my (Ferrell) earliest hospice "teachers" was a young woman who was dying of ovarian cancer and leaving behind a loving husband and two beautiful children. This family was very involved in a fundamentalist Christian church and they were greatly comforted by the support of their church. This patient spoke of the pain of knowing she was leaving her children without a mother, yet she was confident that they would remember her as a model of "what a good Christian woman should be." As a new hospice nurse, I was still struggling with how I could "fix" things in a situation to make things "better" and to "do" for this family rather than "be with" them on this journey. One day I arrived for my visit and found the patient alone and eagerly waiting for me. I was ready—ready to "do" all the things I thought would be important, such as assess her pain, talk with her about her death, or offer to bathe her or wash her beautiful hair. Instead, when I asked her what I could do, she asked if I could go outside and plant tulip bulbs! I was taken off guard by this request. Planting tulips wasn't quite in my job description or on my "list" of what I thought hospice nurses did. The patient explained that each year she planted tulips and that her children loved to see them bloom in the spring and that while she was unable to go outside or kneel on the ground, if I could do this she knew her children would be so comforted when the tulips bloomed and they would know she was thinking of them from heaven. That day, I planted tulips, occasionally pausing to look behind me at my teacher watching carefully through the window

Historical Perspectives

Historically, spirituality was an integral part of the mission and practice of health care institutions and providers. The medical model of practice in healing prior to the 1900s was service-oriented compassionate care. Medical care was primarily supportive and palliative, with limited options for curing disease. Healers utilized a holistic approach of physical, psychological, social, and spiritual care. The first hospitals in the United States were started by religious and service organizations whose service and calling were manifest in a focus of care on the whole person. Men and women choose careers in the health care professions out of a calling to care for others, a desire to serve, and a commitment to make a difference in the patients' well-being (Puchalski & Lunsford, 2006).

With the development of technology in the twentieth century, a biomedical model emerged that focused on "cure" as the leading practice in the view of the western world. The philosophy of present medicine began with René Descartes in the nineteenth century. Descartes alleged that the world operated according to mechanical laws without mention to meaning and purpose. In medicine, Flexner (1910) reported that there was no evidence to support the connection of religion and health. As a result, discussion of spirituality and religion fell out of favor in the study and practice of medicine (Sulmasy, 2006).

In the second half of the twentieth century, there was a resurgence in the interest in spirituality and holistic care with the advent of the religious healing practices, as well as mind-body and integrative practices. Studies that demonstrated an association between spirituality and health triggered the field of medicine to begin to explore the importance of this area in the care of patients. Also, in the latter part of the twentieth century, hospice care became a movement based on the awareness that healing is not just about cure and that people with chronic illness and those facing death could be healed even in the absence of a curative intervention. This healing stemmed from the internal work by the patient to deal with fundamentally spiritual issues about meaning, purpose, and suffering. Healing manifested as transcending the suffering to a place of acceptance of one's finitude.

Biomedical science alone often is focused on cure or fixing an identified problem. In general in palliative care, many problems cannot be fixed or cured, but there is always an opportunity for healing. Healing encourages the patient to focus on finding meaning and hope even in the midst of dying. "Fixing" is the result of training in a biomedical model and facing the limitations of medicine can lead to a loss of hope for clinicians who strive always to fix illness and suffering. But it can also lead to a frustration for the patient as his or her focus also becomes the fix and not the broader concept of healing. Samuel was a bright, accomplished surgical resident in otolaryngology. His patient was a young woman diagnosed with an aggressive facial cancer. Surgery had the potential to give her additional years. Katie asked Samuel, "At what cost? ... So I would look like a monster and die anyway." Samuel responded, "But in the few years that you live longer, we may find a cure." Katie responded, "You don't understand. I can't live that way with half my face removed. I am at peace with dying. Just let me go home and be with my family." Over the next few months, Katie suffered deeply due to the sadness of leaving her husband, her children, and grieving the loss of dreams and hopes. She asked the chaplain, "Why me?" Over time together with her family and the hospice chaplain, Katie was able to surrender to life's seeming injustices and accept not having an answer to the whys. Instead, she rested in the love of her family and her belief that somehow she would be a part of their lives forever.

Spiritual pain cannot be fixed in the way that physical pain can; however, the willingness and ability to facilitate or provide spiritual care ameliorates the frustration frequently experienced when physical care alone can no longer alleviate suffering. An example of this conflict of goals of healing versus fixing was evident in the case of Gladys, an elderly woman with end-stage renal disease. Gladys had enjoyed a life "full to the brim" and with great joy. Her own mother had lived to be 102 and Gladys was shocked to learn that she had advanced renal disease. Her physician had cared for her for thirty years and had treated many "fixable" problems. However, as her renal disease progressed, she required dialysis. While she resisted, her physician insisted that this was the only option. Over the course of the next year, Gladys' life was consumed with dialysis three times per week, multiple doctor visits, frequent lab work, and several acute hospital admissions. Gladys and her very supportive son scheduled a meeting with the doctor to discuss her wish to stop dialysis, knowing she would likely die within a few days, as she had come to the point of believing her quality of life was unacceptable. Her physician initially opposed this request, immediately talking of all the things that could be done, when Gladys interrupted to say, "But I am done." The physician then listened to her request and Gladys was admitted to an inpatient hospice unit, where she spent her final two weeks enjoying visits from family and friends while receiving all the benefits of interdisciplinary care by the hospice social worker, chaplain, and nurses.

In addition to medicine, the field of psychology also contributed to the dissociation of spirituality from health. For decades, there has been a complex relationship between psychology and spirituality that has generated a progressive disconnection between the two disciplines, resulting in a general avoidance of spiritual and religious issues in mainstream psychology. The historical reasons for this disconnect can be traced to the development of modern psychology during the nineteenth and twentieth centuries, a time characterized by the resurgence of scientific discipline and its efforts to challenge religious authority as the source of truth (Barbour, 1990; Hearnshaw, 1987; Hesse, 1980; Lucas, 1985). The assumptions of reductionism, materialism, and empiricism came to dominate the philosophic discourse and were accepted by Freud and the psychoanalytic movement, as well as the behaviorist tradition that followed (Karier, 1986). The "Zeitgeist" or spirit of the time is well reflected in Watson's (1919) comment: "Psychology, up to very recent times, has been held so rigidly under the dominance of both religion and of philosophy—the two great bulwarks of medievalism—that it has never been able to free itself and become a natural science."

However, there have been powerful dissenting voices, such as Jung and Adler. They increasingly criticized the dogmatic rejection of mental processes in favor of the study of consciousness, which opened up the link to spirituality (Yalom, 1980). Spirituality and religion started to be recognized as vehicles adopted by many human beings to make sense of the world, maintain well-being, and achieve self-realization (May, 1969). Psychologists in the 1960s began to research the effect of religion on mental health. This work affected the current reconnection of spirituality in health by providing data that supported some connection between religion and mental health (Koenig et al., 1998). While the data are indicative of the connection, there remains some controversy about the full integration of spirituality into mental health care and health care in general. But it is recognized that these dimensions of human experience can no longer be ignored, and practical steps toward integrating psychological and spiritual dimensions are needed for patient care (Bergin, 1991; Shafranske, 1996).

Of all the models of care in medicine, nursing, psychology, and others, hospice and palliative care most often recognize the importance of spiritual issues in the care of patients and their families. Cecily Saunders recognized the importance of holistic care and developed the biopsychosocial-spiritual model for hospice and palliative care (Sulmasy, 2002; Wald, 1998). Saunders was the first to address spiritual pain of the patient. The National Consensus Project (NCP) Guidelines for Quality Palliative Care (2004) provided recommendations about all domains of care, including the spiritual domain, which is recognized as a critical component of care. Yet the spiritual dimension often receives less emphasis than the biopsychosocial dimensions of care. Spiritual issues are often underrepresented in the literature, including research-based articles related to palliative care (Puchalski et al., 2003). In a recent study by Balboni et al. (2007), 88 percent of patients with terminal cancer found spiritual and religious beliefs to be important in their coping with their illness and dying, yet only 26 percent of those patients felt those needs were met by their medical communities and only 51 percent of those patients felt that their spiritual needs were met by their religious communities. There are many reasons for this, including lack of time in the clinical environment, no training in spiritual care, and fear of offending a patient with seemingly personal questions. Sometimes clinicians say they do not want to engage with a patient at a deeper level, fearing that the patients will share more information than they will have time or skill to deal with in the clinical setting. Yet studies reveal that spiritual or religious beliefs can impact the care of patients in many ways. Spiritual care can impact how patients cope with suffering, pain, and compliance. Paraphrasing Rabbi Heschel: to heal a patient, you must first know a patient (Sulmasy, 1999). Knowing the patient is not just understanding the disease mechanisms but understanding the totality of his or her personhood—the psychosocial and spiritual as well as the physical.

Phelps et al. (2009) found that positive religious coping in patients with advanced cancer was associated with receipt of intensive life-prolonging medical care near the end of life. There are other studies that indicate that spiritual and religious beliefs can impact many health care decisions around treatment. In addition, there is some anecdotal evidence that religion can impact compliance. I (Puchalski) had a patient who was diagnosed with HIV. She refused medications, stating that she had an abortion when she was thirteen after being raped. She noted that the HIV illness was her "punishment from God" and therefore she did not deserve to get better. Gradually, over time and with the help of a chaplain, she forgave herself and was able to accept treatment, treatment she might not have accepted if I had not addressed the spiritual aspect in her care. There is therefore a clear need for our health care systems, particularly those settings where palliative care is practiced, to integrate spiritual care more fully. This book provides recommendations, resources, and tools for health care professionals to support the implementation of the NCP guidelines and National Quality Forum (NQF) preferred practices to better meet the spiritual needs of patients and families.

2 Guidelines/Preferred Practices for Spiritual Care

The National Consensus Project for Quality Palliative Care

The first national guidelines in the United States for palliative care were released in 2004 and revised in 2009 by the National Consensus Project (NCP) for Quality Palliative Care. The purpose of the NCP was to establish clinical practice guidelines that promote consistent and high-quality care and guide the development and structure of new and existing palliative care services. These guidelines are applicable to specialist-level palliative care delivered in a range of treatment settings (e.g., palliative care teams) and to the work of providers in primary treatment settings where palliative approaches to care are integrated into daily clinical practice (e.g., oncology, critical care, long-term care). The NCP guidelines and later the NQF preferred practices were created in recognition of the rapidly expanding field of palliative care. Both the NCP and NQF recognized that palliative care is, by its essence, whole-person care encompassing all dimensions, including spiritual care.

The five leading palliative care organizations participating in the NCP and release of the guidelines were the American Academy of Hospice and Palliative Medicine, the Center to Advance Palliative Care, Hospice and Palliative Nurses Association, Last Acts Partnership, and the National Hospice and Palliative Care Organization. The Last Acts Partnership ended its operation in fall 2004, but the other organizations continue to collaborate. The full guidelines are available at www.nationalconsensusproject.org.

The NCP guidelines were developed through a two-year consensus process, including a review of more than two thousand citations from the literature, a review of thirty-one consensus documents and standards, and peer review by more than two hundred interdisciplinary experts representing diverse settings. The guidelines domain serves as a framework for advancing research and for this book. The purposes of these Clinical Practice Guidelines for Quality Palliative Care are to:

1. Facilitate the development and continuing improvement of clinical palliative care programs providing care to patients and families with life-threatening or debilitating illness.
2. Establish uniformly accepted definitions of the essential elements in palliative care that promote quality, consistency, and reliability of these services.
3. Establish national goals for access to quality palliative care.
4. Foster performance measurement and quality improvement initiatives in palliative care services.

The guideline domains include:

Domain 1: Structure and Processes of Care
Domain 2: Physical Aspects of Care
Domain 3: Psychological and Psychiatric Aspects of Care
Domain 4: Social Aspects of Care
Domain 5: Spiritual, Religious, and Existential Aspects of Care
Domain 6: Cultural Aspects of Care
Domain 7: Care of the Imminently Dying Patient
Domain 8: Ethical and Legal Aspects of Care

While spiritual care is a distinct domain, spiritual and existential concerns are mentioned throughout the guidelines—for example, as aspects of pain, psychological concerns, and grief. Spirituality is clearly a dimension of each domain.

National Quality Forum

The successful dissemination of the NCP guidelines led to the next advancement through collaboration with the National Quality Forum (NQF). Building on the NCP guidelines, in 2006 the NQF released a set of preferred practices for palliative care. The NQF framework was a major advance for the field of palliative care given the status of NQF as the major private-public partnership in the United States responsible for identifying and approving evidence-based quality measures linked to reimbursement (NQF, 2006).

National Consensus Project Guidelines

National Quality Forum
Preferred Practices

SPIRITUAL DOMAIN

DOMAIN 5:

Guideline 5.1: Spiritual and existential dimensions are assessed and responded to based upon the best available evidence, which is skillfully and systematically applied.
Criteria:

spiritual, religious, and existential aspects of care

PREFERRED PRACTICE 20

The interdisciplinary team includes professionals with skill in assessment of and response to the spiritual and existential issues common to both pediatric and adult patients with life-threatening illnesses and conditions, and their families. These professionals should have education and appropriate training in pastoral care and the spiritual issues evoked by patients and families faced with life-threatening illness.

Develop and document a plan based on assessment of religious, spiritual, and existential concerns using a structured instrument and integrate the information obtained from the assessment into the palliative care plan.

The regular assessment of spiritual and existential concerns is documented. This includes, but is not limited to, life review, assessment of hopes and fears, meaning, purpose, beliefs about afterlife, guilt, forgiveness, and life completion tasks.

PREFERRED PRACTICE 21

Provide information about the availability of spiritual care services and make spiritual care available either through organizational spiritual counseling or through the patient's own clergy relationships.

Whenever possible, a standardized instrument should be used to assess and identify religious or spiritual/existential background, preferences, and related beliefs, rituals, and practices of the patient and family.

Periodic reevaluation of the impact of spiritual/existential interventions and patient-family preferences should occur with regularity and be documented. Spiritual/existential care needs, goals, and concerns are addressed and documented, and support is offered for issues of life completion in a manner consistent with the individual's and family's cultural and religious values.

PREFERRED PRACTICE 22

Specialized palliative and hospice care teams should include spiritual care professionals appropriately trained and certified in palliative care.

Pastoral care and other palliative-care professionals facilitate contacts with spiritual/religious communities, groups, or individuals, as desired by the patient and/or family. Of primary importance is that patients have access to clergy in their own religious traditions.

PREFERRED PRACTICE 23

Specialized palliative and hospice spiritual care professionals should build partnerships with community clergy and provide education and counseling related to end-of-life care.

Professional and institutional use of religious/spiritual symbols is sensitive to cultural and religious diversity.

The patient and family are encouraged to display their own religious/spiritual or cultural symbols.

The palliative care service facilitates religious or spiritual rituals or practices as desired by patient and family, especially at the time of death.

Referrals to professionals with specialized knowledge or skills in spiritual and existential issues are made when appropriate.

The NQF is a nonprofit organization whose mission is developing ways to improve the quality of American health care. The NQF endorses consensus-based national standards for measurement and public reporting of health care performance data to direct care that is safe, timely, beneficial, patient-centered, equitable, and efficient. As a public-private partnership, the NQF has involvement from all parts of the health care system, including national, state, regional, and local organizations representing consumers, public and private purchasers, employers, professionals, organizations, health plans, accrediting bodies, labor unions, and other organizations addressing health care research or quality improvement.

The NQF utilizes a five-step process: consensus standard development, widespread review, member voting and council approval, board of directors' action, and subsequent evaluation. The NQF process often leads to standards appropriate for accreditation or reimbursement. Involvement in the field of palliative care by NQF was a critical step to move these aspects of quality care to the attention of those beyond hospice or palliative care to become the interest of policymakers, guide reimbursement, and advance quality improvement, benchmarking, accreditation, and public reporting.

The NQF also accepted the NCP domains for its framework structure and created preferred practices to operationalize the NCP guidelines and to set the foundation for future measurement of the outcomes of care. These preferred practices are all highly relevant to clinical practice. The NQF framework contains thirty-eight best practices across the eight NCP domains. These practices are evidence-based or endorsed through expert opinion and apply to both hospice and palliative care provided across settings. Table 1 includes a list of the NCP guidelines and the NQF preferred practices relating to the spirituality domain.

Spirituality

Spirituality is a term that refers to many dimensions of a person's life. It has been described as the essence of one's humanity (Frankl, 1963) and how people find a sense of who they are or their personhood. Spirituality can also be understood as one's relationship to a transcendence that for some people might be God and for others might be different concepts of how they see themselves in the world and in relationship to something outside of themselves. Spirituality also has a relational component, as in relation to God or to others.

Amidst the myriad of definitions of spirituality found in the literature (some of which are listed in Appendix A) are some common themes to inform our understanding of this concept. Unruh et al.'s (2002) critical review of definitions of spirituality in diverse professional health care literature identified seven thematic categories: (1) relationship to God, a spiritual being, a higher being, or reality greater than the self; (2) not of the self; (3) transcendence or connectedness unrelated to a belief in a higher being; (4) existential, not of the material world; (5) meaning and purpose in life; (6) life force of the person or integrating aspect of the person; and (7) summative definitions that combined multiple themes.

Mauk and Schmidt (2004) defined spirituality as

> The core of a person's being ... usually conceptualized as a "higher" experience or transcendence of oneself. Often, such an experience involves a perception of a personal relationship with a supreme being (such as God). However, many who consider themselves spiritual deny such identification with a higher power. Spirituality, then, also encompasses feelings and thoughts that bring meaning and purpose to human existence or to one's life journey. (p. 2)

A qualitative study conducted by Chao et al. (2002) examining the essence of spirituality in a sample of terminally ill Buddhist and Christian patients (n=6) identified four broad thematic areas: (1) communion with self (self-identity, wholeness, inner peace); (2) communion with others (love, reconciliation); (3) communion with nature (inspiration, creativity); and (4) communion with a higher being (faithfulness, hope, gratitude). These findings are consistent with Burkhardt and Nagai-Jacobson's (2000) observation that "spirituality is known and experienced in relationships" (p. 95). The notions of communion and connectedness underscore the importance of "relationship" in the spiritual well-being of patients and the salience of spiritual care interventions that promote such connectedness.

Spirituality and Religion

The term "spirituality" is sometimes used synonymously with "religion" (Mauk & Schmidt, 2004). Religion is typically equated with an organized system of beliefs, rituals, and practices with which an individual identifies and associates and includes a relationship with a divine being. Religion may or may not be part of a person's spirituality (Smith, 2006). Religion has both a communal and external aspect and an intrinsic aspect that is spirituality. The word "religion" comes from the Latin term *religare* from *re*—again and *ligare*—to bind. Thus, religions talk of spiritual experiences as the rebinding to God. Judaism and mystical Christianity both speak of the "spark of the Divine" in each person (Levine, 2001; Curtsinger & Pierini, 1991).

Clinicians need to be aware of these related concepts because of the relative importance each may play in the lives of their patients. For example, research reviewed by Marler and Hadaway (2002) indicated that some patients see themselves as both spiritual and religious. Other patients who are religious may express their spirituality through identification and involvement within a particular religion. Other patients may claim to be highly spiritual, yet not religious. For these individuals, an important common denominator appears to be the notion of "transcending the commonplace and searching their soul for deeper meaning" (Mauk & Schmidt, 2004, p. 3). Religion is a way people may transcend the commonplace and search for meaning; this might be seen as intrinsic religiosity. Spirituality is the broader umbrella of all people searching for meaning, the sacred or holy in their lives, whether religious or not. Not all patients relate to the concept of spirituality or religion. Some might speak more in philosophical or existential terms. One of my (Puchalski) patients, an advocate for the homeless, suffered a serious stroke, leaving her paralyzed on the right side as well as having some cognitive impairment. She described herself to me as a "card-carrying atheist." When I asked her what gave her significant meaning in her life, she said, "Oh, that's what you mean by spiritual. In that case, it's my work. I spent sixty years of my life serving others, finding shelter for those who had no homes. That was the source of my life, the purpose of it all—now look at me, I have no meaning anymore." The medical student shadowing me in a discussion with this patient said, "I guess she's not spiritual. She has no religion." Yet Sandra's life was highly spiritual, a life full of love and service to others.

I sent the student back in to learn more about Sandra. Two weeks later when she returned to clinic, Chad asked to see her again. When he came out of the room, he was inspired and transformed by Sandra's story. He had decided to volunteer with the homeless. Chad had learned a fuller concept of spirituality from Sandra; Sandra found new meaning in teaching younger people about her passion. It is therefore important to assess patients' spiritual or religious needs and to keep in mind that spirituality is broadly defined, which might include relationships, values, or nature. As an example, an elderly farmer was admitted to a long-term care setting six months after his wife died and his own end-stage pulmonary disease had progressed to the point that he was confined to bed. As his status declined and death seemed likely in a few days, the hospital staff asked if he would like to see a chaplain. The patient politely declined, saying he had "never been a religious man." An astute nurse took the time to ask if there was anything else he would like to do or anything that would be meaningful. The farmer began to weep and said that he would like to "feel the sun on his face and dirt in his hands." With the help of a hospital volunteer, the patient was taken by wheelchair outside the following afternoon, where he sat in the sun and was able to touch the dirt and feel the breeze, all deeply spiritual experiences for this man at life's end.

Spirituality: A Clinical Definition

A definition of spirituality was derived by a consensus conference of clinicians, medical educators, and chaplains (AAMC, 1999) for medical school courses on spirituality and health. Central to this definition is that spirituality has to do with an individual's search for ultimate meaning in life through participation in religion, through relationships with God or a higher power, through family, or as expressed in nature, rationalism, humanism, or the arts. All these factors can influence how patients and health care professionals perceive health and illness and how we interact with one another (AAMC, 1999). Thus, the definition includes a personal expression of spirituality and also a relational one to others. Spirituality therefore is defined not only by meaning and purpose, but also by the connection to self/others/God or a higher power.

Spirituality is broader than religion; in listening for spiritual or existential themes from patients, it is important to recognize that spirituality can be expressed in many different ways. For some patients, church is the spiritual community, while for others it may be friends or family. Spiritual practices may include prayer, meditation, walking in the woods, listening to music or painting, journaling, intentional appreciation of beauty, or being present to the world or others. For some, service to others or professional work is a spiritual practice. For many, values and ways of living become their spiritual practice, such as intentionally doing good works, or striving to make a difference in the world.

There is often a question as to the distinction between spiritual and other psychosocial support. Spiritual care refers to issues of ultimate meaning, values, and relationship with a higher power or the transcendent or sacred. Psychosocial care refers more to issues of emotions and to human relationships. These boundaries are not absolute. For example, there are spiritual dimensions to people's relationships with each other. Hope may be both spiritual and emotional components. Demoralization is an example of a clinical syndrome that has elements of both spiritual and emotional domains. Demoralization syndrome is defined as "a psychiatric state in which hopelessness, helplessness, meaninglessness, and existential distress are the core phenomena" (Kissane et al., 2001). Demoralized patients may present as if they are depressed, but they may not necessarily have clinical depression. Thus, demoralization might be considered a spiritual syndrome.

Demoralization has been differentiated from depression as related to meaninglessness but not having the clinical features of depression (de Figueiredo, 1993). Demoralization becomes a morbid mental state with features of clinical depression when its distress is persistent rather than transient, with the potential to want to give up on life and desire death (Kissane et al., 2001). The approach to simple demoralization might be a spiritual one; the approach to the patient with morbid demoralization would be both spiritual and emotional or psychiatric, treating both the spiritual despair and the clinical depression.

Challenges in Defining Spirituality: Definitions for the Consensus Document

The challenge in defining spirituality is that any definition does not give justice to the full complexity of the human spirit and of the transcendent, however it is understood. Consequently, it becomes difficult to study spirituality and find reductionistic methods for integrating spirituality into health care. During the consensus conference held in February 2009, the interdisciplinary group of participants debated and discussed a definition of spirituality and through a consensus process arrived at the following definition: "Spirituality is the aspect of humanity that refers to the way individuals seek and express meaning and purpose, and the way they experience their connectedness to the moment, to self, to others, to nature and to the significant or sacred."

The conference participants agreed that this definition applied to spiritual care in palliative care and also to care in general. The key concepts in this definition are that spirituality is common to all people and, as Frankl (1963) wrote, the essence of one's humanity. It is that part of people that seeks meaning and purpose in life. This definition also acknowledges the relational aspect of spirituality—the connection to the transcendent, however the person sees it—the significant experience or the sacred, which could be religious or nonreligious. Relationship also extends to other people, as well as one's inner self and to nature.

This definition is used throughout this book for the spiritual care recommendations and recommendations for research. We suggest that this definition be universally adopted for research in spiritual care in palliative care and in health care in general to help standardize the research and literature in this field.

Death is integral to the human mystery. The fact that we die is obvious. Why we must die and what happens to us after death are questions that have no empirical answers. Yet these questions arise inevitably for creatures that are conscious of their own mortality. Religions have addressed the mystery of death from before the time of recorded history. The practice of burying the dead, accompanied by ritual, dates back tens of thousands of years. Prehistoric passage tombs, such as the one at Newgrange, Ireland, are believed to have been sites for religious rituals of death and rebirth, celebrated in connection with the winter solstice. The Egyptian practices of mummification and the construction of the pyramids all relate to rituals of death and afterlife. Cremation arose contemporaneously in both the East and the West almost five thousand years ago and has persisted as the religiously normative ritual in the East.

Rituals and religious practices also arose early in history among those who anticipated their own deaths or the deaths of those they loved. Dying persons prepared spiritually for death. Even today there are many cultures throughout the world that utilize ritual to step into the profound experience of illness and end of life. Although these rituals are often connected to religious practice, they are at the same time intrinsically part of cultural values and norms as well. We possess a rich and fertile history of how to care for each other in this time of change and ultimate transition. For many communities, death is something seen every day and the health of the community depends on how the village comes together to acknowledge and grieve as a whole. One can say that deep down we know how to care for each other in these moments, because we have been doing it for a very long time.

Most of the major religions address spiritual preparation for death. In the Hebrew Scriptures, several chapters (47–50) of the Book of Genesis are devoted to describing the spiritual aspects of Jacob's final days.

This passage begins with Jacob (Israel), conscious of his impending death, aware that he was at the beginning of the end of his spiritual journey on earth. His acts ritually recall those of his grandfather Abraham. The text describes how Jacob gathers his family, prays aloud, and blesses each of his sons. Maimonides wrote that illness is sickness of the soul, and that in order to heal the body, the soul must be healed (Levine, 2001). To this day Orthodox Jews are encouraged to recite psalms as death approaches, pray the confessional prayer of Yom Kippur—called Vidui—and recite the Shema ("Hear O Israel, the Lord is our God, the Lord is One . . .") from Deuteronomy (6:4). If the sick person is very near to death (*a goses*), or is otherwise unable to pray, friends and relatives are encouraged to recite these prayers on behalf of the dying person.

In his Long Rules, written for monks in the fourth century, St. Basil of Caesarea instructed the monks never to neglect the care of their souls as they prepared for death, regardless of their use of the medical arts. In the Middle Ages, the practice of the *ars moriendi* ("the art of dying well") became a cultural norm for lay persons as well. It was not uncommon for monks as they passed each other in the monastery halls to say *momento mori*, "remember death." Christian men and women who knew they were dying read particular spiritual writings, attempted to make amends with those they had wronged, and tried to cultivate an attitude of calm and faith in God's mercy. It was also important that they confessed their sins and received the sacraments of the anointing of the sick and viaticum (the last communion, literally "food for the journey"). Within these rituals is the deep sacrifice and transformation of Christ, which possesses within it the hope for the soul to be restored and healed through divine grace.

Islamic tradition sees life and the body as a "tenant in this temple (i.e., the human body) for Him who made him to dwell therein and stipulated that in lieu of the payment of rent for his dwelling, he take care of its upkeep and preservation, its cleaning, repair, and use in a manner that would help him in his search for happiness in both this world and the next world" (Sachedina, 2005). Therefore the care of the body throughout this life is important, and care is especially taken at the time of death. As with the other traditions, certain prayers are said and a ritual washing of the body is performed. This is done with care and respect, and when the body is buried, it is oriented in the direction of Mecca.

For Hinduism, in the Bhagavad Gita it is written, "On whatever sphere of being the mind of man may be intent at the time of death, thither will he go" (Sivananda, 2000). There is a practical understanding of the nature of death and a clear awareness that our lives are fragile. Hindus believe in the notion that we have done this living over and over for many lifetimes and in many forms. Therefore if we are not careful, we can affect the next life with the actions of this one. Our state of mind plays a part to our ability to change the future. Important as well is the realization that suffering has its own rules. "One who is free from sin suffers calamities, while sinners are living happily. A rich man dies young and a poor fellow drags on his existence, weighed down by decrepitude. All this is the work of destiny" (*Mahabharata* 12.28). There is no predicting the "why," just that we must know that it is.

Buddhism, which grew from the Hindu tradition, took these messages to heart by making them foundational to the development of the Buddhist philosophy. For young Prince Siddhartha, it was the very vision of old age, sickness, and death that compelled him to transform his life into the path of spiritual practice. It is why the act of attending to someone who is dying is considered one of the most profound lessons one can experience. For many in the Buddhist tradition, it can be a time of great peace and clarity. It is also a time when the environment created around the person is one that emphasizes practice. This often includes chanting, meditation, and at times particular practices designed to support the person as he or she transitions from one life to the next. Perhaps one of the best examples of these particular approaches is *The Tibetan Book of the Dead* (Evans-Wentz, 1927), known traditionally as the *Bardo Thodol*, and first translated in 1927. This thousand-year-old text is an example of the intricate and detailed approach to the act of dying that Buddhism has become known for. There is an encouragement here to turn toward our experience, whatever it may be, so that we may know it more deeply and without fear. From here, we can truly be in peace (Padmasambhava, 2005).

Although these great religions of the world still continue in their concern for those who are seriously ill and dying, more recent decades have witnessed a falling away of spiritual care and religious practices for the dying. This has been particularly true in the West. One reason for this has been a decline in overt religious affiliation and practice. Another reason, for better or worse, may be the translocation of the care of the dying from the home to the hospital. We see this borne out in the fact that even today over 70 percent of the population still dies in an inpatient setting. Slowly, the dying have found themselves physically distanced from their families and communities of faith. The power of the modern hospital has amplified the troubles caused by this translocation. Hospitals focus on saving lives, not always assuring that they end peacefully. And even if family and clergy were to visit, the technology interferes by erecting further barriers—ventilators, dialysis machines, isolation rooms, gowns, and gloves. The goal of hospice and palliative care is to humanize hospital and long-term care settings so that patients and families can find a place to rest, reflect, and be more intentional in the way they face their dying, surrounded by love and compassion. And even in situations when cure is being sought, the issues of quality of life have the same importance as the delivery of technical intervention. One of us (Puchalski) has been working with hospitals to create healing environments through the introduction of spiritual intervention (Puchalski & McSkimming, 2006). Patients, family, and caregivers note greater satisfaction with care and a greater sense of compassion in their caregivers. This book presents a model for interprofessional care that increases spiritual awareness in patient care.

Lost spiritual opportunities have pressed deeply upon the psyches of many who have lost loved ones in settings that seem to deny the reality and inevitability of death. A central motivation for the initiation of the modern hospice movement in the mid- to late twentieth century was the need to reintegrate spirituality into the care of others. Since that time, there has been an ongoing presence of spiritual care within the hospice movement, with a striving for professional practice that is more integrated and rooted in the work of the heart. Chaplains, as professional spiritual care providers, have always had an integral role in the hospice team. For all health care professionals there has been an encouragement toward understanding our personal spiritual values and how those affect our work and care.

Death is as mysterious now as it has always been. There are no empirical answers to questions about the meaning and purpose of human life and death. Spirituality remains as important a part of the dying process in the twenty-first century as it was thousands of years ago. Yet clearly there are modern challenges to maintaining the foundational elements of care that were developed long ago. Technology has made the task of dying complex and seemingly within our control. Science- and technology-driven health care systems do not often offer the space, time, and opportunity for people to struggle with the deep spiritual questions that often arise.

Philosophical and Ethical Issues

A call for health care professionals to engage in spiritual care for patients at the end of life raises moral questions for many. How can one justify a significant departure from decades of a purely scientifically based medical practice? Why should social workers, physicians, nurses, and other health care providers be involved? How could such a practice be contemplated in an increasingly religiously pluralistic society? Such questions require answers.

Some have tried to ground the moral warrant for clinicians to become involved in the spiritual care of patients on empirical data, citing research demonstrating that many patients (a majority in most surveys) want their physicians and nurses to address spiritual issues with them. However, these data do not constitute a sufficient moral warrant to justify clinicians engaging in spiritual care. It is a *necessary* moral condition that a patient consent to an intervention by a clinician, but a patient's preference for an intervention is not *sufficient* as a moral warrant. For example, the bare fact that a patient desires to be treated with hyperbaric oxygen as a remedy for depression is not a sufficient moral justification for a physician to prescribe this treatment.

Nor are data demonstrating an association between patient spiritual practices and salutary health care outcomes a moral warrant for spiritual interventions by clinicians. This is not because these data are invalid. Several long-term epidemiologic studies (Gillum et al., 2008), controlling carefully for many possible confounding factors, have established that, independent of denomination, those who attend religious services on a regular basis live longer than those who do not.

Religious practices and attitudes have also been associated with better mental health outcomes (McCauley et al., 2008). However, these data do not establish that it is religion per se that brings these health benefits. These effects could be mediated through a complex mixture of "secular" explanations (e.g., social support, stress reduction). All that has been established by these retrospective studies is an association, and the only real proof would require a randomized controlled trial assigning half the patients to religious belief and practice and the other half to some sort of secular meditation and support group. Such a trial, of course, would be unethical and absurd.

Such data could not, in principle, constitute a moral warrant to "prescribe" religion the way a physician might "prescribe" regular physical exercise. While these data associating good health outcomes with religious practice might be true, (a) there is no definitive causal proof that religious practice per se improves health outcomes, (b) attending religious services for the "extrinsic" reason of improving health might not confer the health benefits because they might only be associated with "intrinsic" religiosity, and (c) on purely religious grounds, no pastor would want a congregation filled with people who were there only for the health benefits. Authentic religious practice requires a commitment of one's whole person—heart, mind, body, and soul—in a manner more akin to marriage than to exercise. This marks a profound moral difference. While it is true that married people live longer, a physician is not justified urging a single patient to become married "for the health benefits."

Nor is it even necessary, on religious or secular grounds, that religiosity be associated with improved health outcomes in order to justify clinical attention to the spiritual needs of patients. This is because spirituality's role in human experience is more concerned with process and presence than it is with outcomes. From a spiritual point of view, better health is not the goal of spirituality. Spirituality concerns a person's relationship with transcendence. The primary spiritual questions are truly universal and comprise questions of meaning, value, and relationship. Questions such as "Why me?" or "Is there any meaning in what I suffer?" or "Do I still have value now that illness has rendered me unproductive?" or "Am I really loved?" or "Can I bring myself to forgive those who have wronged me?" are the sorts of spiritual interrogatives that arise spontaneously and ubiquitously in the experiences of illness, injury, and death. Spirituality is concerned with how one lives one's life and experiences death in light of whether one sees answers to these questions that transcend the finitude of human space and time.

Physicians, nurses, and other health care professionals commit themselves, often by oath, to caring for patients as whole persons. Because illness and injury disrupt a patient's life in ways that extend beyond the body, encompassing families, communities, and a patient's religious commitments, a commitment to caring for whole persons must entail going beyond the care of only the body. A human being is a spiritual being. When injured or ill, human beings naturally ask transcendent questions about meaning, value, and relationship. If providing holistic care is a moral duty, then that duty extends to the spiritual as well as to the physical. Therefore, attending to the spiritual needs of patients is not just a moral option, it constitutes a moral imperative. Attending to the spiritual needs of patients is justified because spirituality is intrinsic to the nature of being sick and caring for the sick. This imperative is only amplified by the existential predicament of the patient at the end of life.

Each of the health care professions has in its professional code standards that relate to the provision of compassionate care and for addressing spirituality with patients and families.

Medicine

Guidelines from several organizations, including the American College of Physicians (ACP, 2009) and The Joint Commission (2008), recognize the need for spiritual care. An ACP consensus conference on end-of-life care concluded that physicians have the obligation to address all dimensions of suffering, including spiritual, religious, and existential suffering. The conference also developed guidelines for communicating with patients about spiritual and religious matters (Lo et al., 1999). The Joint Commission requires that spiritual care be available to patients in hospital settings. A consensus conference cosponsored by the Association of American Medical Colleges and the George Washington Institute for Spirituality and Health also developed guidelines for spiritual care (Puchalski et al., 2004).

In addition, theoretical and ethical frameworks, upon which health care professional education and practice is built, include spirituality as an essential aspect of competent health care of patients, including the biopsychosocial-spiritual model, that recognizes that patients experience health and illness in many dimensions (Sulmasy, 2002). This model is the basis of palliative care and hospice, which recognizes the psychosocial and spiritual aspects of patients and families as well as the physical. The Institute of Medicine (IOM, 2001) describes patient-centered care as a critical element of high-quality health care that improves the safety and efficacy of patient care. Patient-centered care is important for its shared decision making, respect for patients' values and beliefs, involvement of a larger community of caregivers, and increased safety of care (Institute for Alternative Futures, 2004). Shared decision making requires knowledge of the factors affecting a patient's decision-making process, which include spiritual, religious, and cultural beliefs. It also includes spiritual beliefs and values that can affect decision making and the patient's ability to cope with illness and find hope in the midst of suffering.

Nursing

Nursing theories include aspects of spirituality in patient care, directly or indirectly, including caring (Watson, 1999), interpersonal relationships, and spiritual variables (Neuman, 1995). One of six essential features of professional nursing practice is the establishment of a caring relationship to facilitate health and healing (American Nurses Association, 2003). Spirituality has actually been described as the "cornerstone of holistic nursing practice" (Nagai-Jacobson & Burkhardt, 1989) and as "the integrating aspect of human wholeness ... integral to quality care" (Clark et al., 1991). Nurses apply scientific knowledge to the process of diagnosis and treatment of total human responses to health and illness, such as alteration in bowel function, hopelessness, and alteration in nutrition. In 1978, the first nursing diagnosis related to spirituality, Spiritual Distress, was included in the taxonomy developed by the North American Nursing Diagnosis Association (now NANDA International).

The Code of Ethics for professional nurses in the United States (ANA, 2001) recognizes the importance of spirituality and health, illustrated by provision 1 of the code, which states, "The nurse, in all professional relationships, practices with compassion and respect for the inherent dignity, worth, and uniqueness of each individual, unrestricted by considerations of social and economic status, personal attributes, or the nature of health problems." Interpretive statements for this provision of the code further assert that "the measures nurses take to care for the patients enable the patients to live with as much physical, psychological, social, and spiritual well-being as possible" (provision 1.3). The International Council of Nurses (2006) Code for Nurses states, "The nurse promotes an environment in which the human rights, values, customs and spiritual beliefs of the individual, family and community are respected" (p. 4). Both of these codes highlight the importance of including spiritual care as an essential aspect of competent and compassionate nursing practice. Nurses provide compassionate care and dignity to persons near the end of life because nurses spend more time than any other profession at the bedside and in the community with patients and their families experiencing end-of-life care issues (Ferrell & Coyle, 2006, 2008). Nurses serve as leaders in all clinical settings, on palliative care services, and as parish nurses.

Social Work

The National Association of Social Workers' Code of Ethics (2008) declares that a social worker must include spirituality when completing an assessment. Similar to other professions, social workers are challenged to meet this recommendation due to the lack of available spiritual assessment tools. The six core values of the social work profession from the National Association of Social Workers (NASW) are service, social justice, dignity and worth of the person, importance of human relationships, integrity, and competence. While these are all important, two are of particular importance at the end of life: dignity and worth of the person and the importance of human relationships. Social workers treat each person in a caring and respectful fashion, mindful of individual differences as well as cultural, ethnic, and religious diversity. Social workers promote clients' socially responsible self-determination. Social workers seek to enhance clients' capacity and opportunity to change and address their own needs. Social workers are cognizant of their dual responsibility to clients and to the broader society. They seek to resolve conflicts between clients' interests and the broader society's interests in a socially responsible manner consistent with the values, ethical principles, and ethical standards of the profession.

Social workers understand that relationships between and among people are an important vehicle for change. Social workers engage people as partners in the helping process. Social workers seek to strengthen relationships among people in a purposeful effort to promote, restore, maintain, and enhance the well-being of individuals, families, social groups, organizations, and communities. Within the NASW code, there are several ethical standards that apply, which are listed in table 2.

TABLE 2   Selections from (NASW) Ethical Standards

---

1. Social Workers' Ethical Responsibilities to Clients

1.01	**Commitment to Clients:** Social workers' primary responsibility is to promote the well-being of clients.

1.03	**Informed Consent:** Social workers should provide services to clients only in the context of a professional relationship based, when appropriate, on valid informed consent.

1.05   **Cultural Competence and Social Diversity**

a) Social workers should understand culture and its function in human behavior and society, recognizing the strengths that exist in all cultures.

b) Social workers should have a knowledge base of their clients' cultures and be able to demonstrate competence in the provision of services that are sensitive to clients' cultures and to differences among people and cultural groups.

c) Social workers should obtain education about and seek to understand the nature of social diversity and oppression with respect to race, ethnicity, national origin, color, sex, sexual orientation, gender identity or expression, age, marital status, political belief, religion, immigration status, and mental or physical disability.

2.03   **Interdisciplinary Collaboration**

a) Social workers who are members of an interdisciplinary team should participate in and contribute to decisions that affect the well-being of clients by drawing on the perspectives, values, and experiences of the social work profession. Professional and ethical obligations of the interdisciplinary team as a whole and of its individual members should be clearly established.

2.06   **Referral for Services**

a) Social workers should refer clients to other professionals when the other professionals' specialized knowledge or expertise is needed to serve clients fully or when social workers believe that they are not being effective or making reasonable progress with clients and that additional service is required.

4.01   **Competence**

a) Social workers should accept responsibility or employment only on the basis of existing competence or the intention to acquire the necessary competence.

b) Social workers should strive to become and remain proficient in professional practice and the performance of professional functions. Social workers should critically examine and keep current with emerging knowledge relevant to social work. Social workers should routinely review the professional literature and participate in continuing education relevant to social work practice and social work ethics.

c) Social workers should base practice on recognized knowledge, including empirically based knowledge, relevant to social work and social work ethics.

(National Association of Social Workers, 2008)

Chaplains and Other Spiritual Care Professionals

Spiritual care professionals are trained to work with people of all beliefs and faiths. Their focus is on the spiritual health of individuals and families. They affirm the dignity and value of each individual and respect the right of each faith group to hold its values and traditions. They work with believers and nonbelievers alike.

Spiritual care professionals understand clients to be any patient, family member, student, or staff to whom they provide spiritual care. In these relationships, spiritual care professionals uphold the following standards of professional ethics.

1. Speak and act in ways that honor the dignity and value of every individual.
2. Provide care that is intended to promote the best interest of the client and to offer strength, integrity, and healing.
3. Demonstrate respect for the cultural and religious values of those they serve and refrain from imposing their own values and beliefs on those served. (Canadian Association for Pastoral Practice and Education/Association canadienne pour la practique et l'éducation pastorals, 2008)

Professional chaplains offer spiritual care to all who are in need and have specialized education to mobilize spiritual resources so that patients cope more effectively. They maintain confidentiality and provide a supportive context within which patients can discuss their concerns. They are professionally accountable to their religious faith group, their certifying chaplaincy organization, and the employing institution. Professional chaplains and their certifying organizations demonstrate a deep commitment and sensitivity to the diverse ethnic and religious cultures found in North America (VandeCreek & Burton, 2001).

Psychology

Many psychologists and other mental health and health care professionals believe that addressing spirituality benefits the individual. Addressing spiritual concerns may be therapeutically important for patients' well-being. Accordingly, providing psychotherapy to patients with advanced illness who may be approaching death requires psychologists to be aware of the potential spiritual concerns of advanced illness and death for their patients. This also means psychologists need to screen for and recognize spiritual distress; make appropriate referrals when necessary; and, based on their level of training and experience, explore patient concerns during the therapy session. Psychologists working in the palliative care setting are familiar with the struggle involved in caring for palliative care patients. The ability to identify cognitive, emotional, spiritual, religious, cultural, and social resources that can be mobilized to assist the patient is recognized as an important part of the therapeutic work. Equally important is the ability to identify possible sources of distress that may increase suffering for patients and their caregivers (Richards & Bergin, 2002). Understanding a patient's spiritual and religious orientation, developing an appreciation for how it can support the patient during the difficult journey through illness and death, and correctly identifying possible sources of spiritual or religious distress are part of the important assessment psychologists make in collaboration with the other members of the team. In this important context, spirituality, meaning and purpose, and religiosity cannot dogmatically be conceptualized as outside the boundaries of psychotherapy. Working with palliative-care patients requires psychologists to address spirituality as part of the personal value system shared by the patient and the family.

When describing professional roles for psychologists in end-of-life care, the American Psychological Association (APA, 2002) mentions spiritual and existential concerns as one of the key assessment areas that need to be addressed when working with patients. Recognizing the impact of spirituality on many patients' value systems, psychologists are encouraged to explore this area in order to understand patients' motivations behind difficult requests, including refusal of care, unreasonable intensity of care, and a hastened death.

The most recent ethical guidelines for psychologists published by the APA (2002) explicitly include religion as a type of diversity to which psychologists need to be sensitive. This means religion is recognized to be as important as culture, gender, sexual orientation, and ethnic background in determining patients' understanding of the world, of themselves, and of others. Psychology of Religion, one of the divisions of the APA, promotes the study of the nature and application of religion and spirituality, with the goal of facilitating communication between psychological study and practice and spiritual and religious perspectives and institutions.

Physician Assistants

The American Academy of Physician Assistants' (2008) "Guidelines for Ethical Conduct for the Physician Assistant Profession" clearly states mandates for end-of-life care:

> Among the ethical principles that are fundamental to providing compassionate care at the end of life, the most essential is recognizing that dying is a personal experience and part of the life cycle.... PAs should assure terminally-ill patients that their dignity is a priority and that relief of physical and mental suffering is paramount. PAs should exhibit non-judgmental attitudes and should assure their terminally-ill patients that they will not be abandoned.... PAs should explain palliative and hospice care and facilitate patient access to those services. End of life care should include assessment and management of psychological, social, and spiritual or religious needs.... While respecting patients' wishes for particular treatments when possible, PAs also must weigh their ethical responsibility, in consultation with supervising physicians, to withhold futile treatments and to help patients understand such medical decisions.

Other

In addition, all members of the transdisciplinary team should have spiritual care experience, education, and training. These include all health care professionals such as physical, occupational, and respiratory therapists; pharmacists; home health aides; clinical nurse assistants; and others. There are also unlicensed health care providers that are integral to the care of patients and may also participate in the overall patient-centered approach to care, including spiritual care.

Ethical Issues in Providing Spiritual Care

Ethical Guidelines

While advocating that clinicians should become engaged in attending to the spiritual needs of patients, we recognize that certain special characteristics of the relationship between a clinician and a patient help shape how this is carried out in practice. The first important characteristic to note is the marked power imbalance between the clinician and the patient. The sick, and especially those who are dying, often have little of the normal control that most human beings have over their lives. They may be weak. They may have impaired decision-making capacity. They do not exercise command over the powerful information needed to diagnose and treat themselves. All of this power and control belongs to the clinician, who must be careful to never exploit a patient in his or her weakness, vulnerability, and diminished personal autonomy. Clinicians have a profound moral obligation to be trustworthy and to use their power in the interests of their patients. Second, there is a deep intimacy in the spiritual domain. Spirituality is an aspect of life that is close to the core of a person. To have access to the intimate aspects of a person's life demands that the one granted such access exercise care, restraint, and confidentiality. Third, it is important to point out that while spiritual concerns can assume a particular salience at the end of life, attention to the spiritual needs of patients is not just something to be reserved for care as patients approach death. Spiritual needs are intrinsic to the human experience of illness and injury and it would be a mistake to limit attention to patients' spiritual needs solely at the end of life. An example of the need to incorporate spiritual care for all patients is evident in the field of oncology. Each year, over 1.5 million people are diagnosed with cancer and many of these will be successfully treated. In fact, there are over 12 million cancer survivors living in the United States today. There is growing evidence in the cancer survivorship literature that can even when long-term survival or cure is possible, once a person hears the words "you have cancer," his or her life is changed forever. Patients diagnosed with cancer need attention to spiritual care regardless of prognosis.

In all matters related to spirituality and health care, the best course is to always follow the patient's lead. Some who are troubled by attention to spiritual needs have based their concerns on worries about issues such as proselytizing by clinicians or the possibility that patients' autonomy might be restricted by the overzealous clinical application of moral views particular to the clinician's personal religion. These sorts of worries are not unfounded, but they can be mitigated significantly by constantly obeying the simple rule of following the patient's lead. Simple inquiries such as "What role, if any, does spirituality or religion play in your life?" or "How are you doing with all this? I mean, with the big questions?" could not reasonably be construed as offensive or attempts to "impose religion on patients." While clinicians are often taught interviewing skills and specific techniques for obtaining information about sensitive topics such as sexual practices or substance abuse, it is far less likely that physicians, nurses, or others entering practice have been taught the language or skills associated with spiritual practice.

What ought to happen next will depend upon the patient's response. Experienced clinicians will know how to proceed based upon the verbal and nonverbal reactions of the patient, who may invite more discussion or not. Some patients may not want to discuss their beliefs. Their privacy should be respected. Questions should also be asked in a manner that conveys openness to all types of beliefs—humanistic, religious, and nontheist alike. Some patients may have had traumatic experiences with religious or spiritual organizations. They may be resistant to disclose their backgrounds. Finally, atheists or nonbelievers may not disclose their beliefs or lack of beliefs. Thus, a spiritual history or assessment must be sensitive enough to identify concerns in all patients and ask general questions that invite all patients to share what is important to them and their care (Bergin, 1991; Bergin & Strupp, 1972; Richards & Bergin, 2002; Strada & Sourkes, 2009; Strada, 2008).

Respect, patient-centeredness, and inclusivity are three key ethical principles that can guide palliative care and general medical care practice (Canda & Furman, 1999; Nelson-Becker et al., 2006). Respect means to value the patient's views even if they seem very different from more frequently encountered belief systems. At this point in his/her course of illness, a patient may not want to hear other views about life beyond death or lack of it. Certainly it is not advisable for a professional to share his or her own beliefs in the hope of changing a patient's view. Respect also extends to the recognition that individuals are unique—two people of the same religious affiliation do not necessarily follow all the dogmas of the religion (Karier, 1986; Maslow, 1962; Watson, 1919; Yalom, 1980).

As much as possible, the patient should be encouraged and empowered to make decisions he or she is able and want to make. Finally, the principle of inclusivity and acceptance encourages professionals to develop a holistic care that invites significant others to be a part of the healing and palliative care medical community.

Boundaries   To have appropriate therapeutic relationships with patients and families, boundaries need to be recognized. Boundaries are mutually understood, unspoken, physical, emotional, social, and spiritual limits of the professional. Where the clinician ends, the other person begins. The clinician-patient relationship is often a one-way relationship that lacks mutuality and reciprocity. Yet there is a significant intimacy in the sharing of a patient's pain, suffering, meaning, and hopes. Thus, there is a need for balance between intimacy and power; boundaries help with that balance.

Boundaries contribute to therapeutic alliance, reduce patient risks from power imbalance, maintain clinician objectivity, promote clinician safety, and protect clinicians' well-being. Boundaries are a healthy recognition of the purpose of the relationship while avoiding putting up walls. Boundaries allow clinicians to be in the present moment with others and passively allow emotional, physical, or social distractions to flow freely, not interrupting the patient-clinician interaction. For example, if the patient verbalizes thoughts that for whatever reason are troublesome for the clinician, recognizing the professional boundary can allow for continuation of the therapeutic relationship by focusing on the therapeutic issue and not the words or the emotions from the patient that could potentially distract the clinician. For example, if a terminally ill patient seeks counseling to discuss his estrangement from his family and reveals that in the past he had abused his former wife, the therapist would need to avoid a personal response to his or her feelings about abuse in order to focus on the current situation and the need to support the patient in seeking forgiveness.

Distancing, which many clinicians use to protect themselves, is based on a fear of entanglement. Distancing is the process some clinicians use to prevent themselves from developing a relationship with the patient. In the process of distancing, the clinician does not allow himself or herself to empathize or connect to the patient's pain or suffering. To patients, a clinician who is distancing appears cold or unfeeling. Jason, a medical resident, took care of an elderly man, Ben, in the hospital. Ben reminded Jason of his own grandfather. Jason spent long hours talking to Ben and even made plans to see Ben at his house after discharge. Jason began to spend less time with other patients in order to visit with Ben. On Ben's second hospital day, his condition worsened. Jason expressed sadness and concern that Ben might die. Jason's own anxiety about Ben dying worsened over the next two days. He finally told his senior resident he needed to "pull back." He started avoiding Ben and only spent a minimal time in Ben's room, doing only the necessary technical care. Had Jason utilized appropriate boundaries, he would not have had to practice distancing. Appropriate boundaries in this case would have resulted in Jason's awareness that Ben reminded him of his grandfather but not an overidentification as demonstrated by his spending long hours with Ben and offering social visits.

As a result, when Ben became ill, Jason reacted as if Ben was his grandfather. A better approach would have been for Jason to have a self-awareness of his responses and modify his behavior accordingly. While seeing Ben as his grandfather, a self-aware Jason would have recognized he was not his grandfather and controlled his overidentification. Then he could have been present to Ben and attentive, but not driven to overattentiveness by his overidentification. When Ben became ill, Jason could express his concern and even feel sadness but not overreact with the same emotions he might have for his grandfather. Jason's lack of awareness and utilization of healthy boundaries resulted in his need to distance—to pull away completely in order to function. Self-awareness training allows clinicians to utilize healthy boundaries in forming professionally intimate relationships with patients that are based on healthy motivations rather than unhealthy hidden drives on the part of the clinician, such as overidentification. Distancing actually jeopardizes the clinical relationship in that it breaks the potential for a compassionate connection. Boundaries allow for compassionate presence in the healing encounter. Establishing professional boundaries sets limits but allows the clinician to remain connected to the patient, recognizing the limits to the therapeutic relationship. Clinicians are more vulnerable to crossing boundaries when they are overworked, stressed, or have experienced losses or grief. It is important for clinicians to have avenues for self-care and reflection.

Specific Ethical Concerns

Prohibition on Proselytizing in the Clinical Setting   For many clinicians, this seems obvious. However, certain clinicians, motivated to proselytize patients by virtue of zealous devotion to their own faith commitments, might not agree. They might ask, for example, "If I have the answer to all human concerns, how can I, morally, not share that with everyone I meet, including my patients?" Those who have an intuitive sense that it is wrong for clinicians to proselytize their patients might also need assistance in understanding exactly why their intuitions are justified.

The power imbalance between clinician and patient and the vulnerability of the patient limit the power of the patient to assent freely to the offer to convert. To the extent that the "conversion" is successful only because the patient fears, whether justifiably or not, a diminution in care, or even a loss of esteem in the eyes of the powerful clinician, such a "conversion" will not be free but coerced and therefore false, and the clinician will have been frustrated in his or her aims. From the viewpoint of religious belief, the attempt to take advantage of the patient's predicament as an "opportunity" for proselytizing is really an act of hubris, usurping a prerogative that belongs properly to God. The believer must suppose that God or a higher being freely gave human beings the gift of freedom and can only really be loved if a person comes to faith wholly and freely. If God risks rejection in order that human love of God be free, a believing clinician cannot justly claim the right to take advantage of a patient's weakness to manipulate an act of faith. The intimacy of religious belief and practice makes religion qualitatively different from other attitudes and behaviors a clinician might suggest to patients, such as exercising regularly and eating a low-fat diet. A clinician is not justified advising patients to "get religion," even if his or her intent is beneficent. Even if a patient were to convert freely after having been proselytized by a physician or nurse, the power imbalance of the clinical relationship suggests that despite a good outcome, the use of the relationship to achieve this end would still make the act morally wrong. Proselytizing within the clinical relationship is always a manipulative and subtly coercive act, taking unfair advantage of the patient's situation. To the extent that the clinician, even subconsciously, derives the personal benefit of self-satisfaction from having "won souls for God," the proselytizing of patients is exploitive.

Encouraging Spirituality for the Health Benefits   Some clinicians wish to encourage spiritual or religious beliefs, attitudes, and practices because of the data suggesting a link between religiosity and health care outcomes. Such data are not a sufficient moral warrant for making such recommendations to patients as discussed in Chapter 4. The data demonstrate associations with health care outcomes but not causal evidence needed to justify any sound medical intervention. It is also possible that no health benefits would accrue to those who seek only an "extrinsic" benefit from religion such as improved health. From a theological perspective, people adhere to religious practices and beliefs from a spiritual motivation, not a utilitarian one where practice is for the sole purpose of health outcomes. From the perspective of faith, God is the ground of medicine, the reason for medicine, and the ultimate end of medicine. Ultimately, it is God's outcome, not the individual's or the clinician's, that prevails.

It is critically important to note, however, that neither the prohibition on proselytizing nor the prohibition on suggesting religious belief and practice to patients should be construed as a prohibition on clinicians asking patients whether they have spiritual or religious beliefs and practices that might be helpful to them in coping with illness or coming to grips with the looming possibility of death. These sorts of questions are not threatening to patients, are not denominationally specific, and do not signal a particular answer the patient can presume the clinician considers "correct." They do open a dialogue that can be tailored to the patient's specific needs. To shun such discussions seems disrespectful to patients and a failure to consider them as whole persons.

Prayer Requests from Patients   Part of spiritual care involves integrating spiritual practices. There have been several surveys that demonstrate a desire by some patients to be able to pray with their physicians and nurses (CBS News/New York Times Poll, 1998). In a study of 157 hospitalized adults, McNeill et al. (1998) found that prayer was the second most common patient-reported way to control pain after pain pills. A study by the National Institute of Complementary and Alternative Medicine showed that prayer is the second most commonly used method that hospitalized patients rely upon for pain control, after opioid analgesics (Barnes et al., 2002). Guidelines on praying with patients have been addressed (Astrow et al., 2001; Lo et al., 2003). In general, a moral position ruling out certain practices in all circumstances, such as the ban we propose on proselytizing, requires a great deal of justification. In most ethical matters, however, it is better to give guidelines about when a certain practice would be required, when it might be permissible, when it would be inadvisable, and when it would be wrong.

Chaplains and clergy have been praying with patients for centuries. Chaplains follow the rule of taking the patient's lead and ought only to pray with patients who have asked for such prayers or have consented to a nonmanipulative invitation to prayer. Chaplains and clergy also have training on how to lead prayers; most clinicians do not have that training. In recognition of the power differential between health care professionals and patients, it is critical that patients trust will not be abused by their health care professionals. Thus, having a health care professional invite patients to pray or lead a prayer for a patient is inappropriate in most situations in the clinical settings. The safest rule is always to follow the patient's lead. Exceptions may include similar faiths of both health care professional and patient or long-standing relationships where the patient has asked the health care professional to lead prayer. Further, in these encounters, both the clinician and the patient must engage in a careful and mutually respectful dialogue, recognizing that both are moral agents and individuals will vary greatly as they "negotiate" a level of comfort. In cases where it's not clear how to best attend to the patients' spiritual needs, the clinicians should refer to the chaplain.

One should keep in mind that patients' requests for prayer usually are rare but also may be a very powerful call to connect with the health care professional. While it is generally recommended that health care professionals not offer prayer, if a patient requests it, the clinician should respond sensitively. Thus, a health care professional who has personal ethics against prayer but is asked by the patient to pray might consider standing by in silence as the patient prays or offering to get a chaplain to lead the prayer. In all interactions, the good of the patient must come first. Imposing the health care professional's belief system or prayer on the patient is not appropriate. But rejecting a request outright without considering other appropriate options for the patient request might similarly adversely affect the patient.

Some patients may still insist on having the physician or nurse lead the prayer. If the clinician is comfortable praying with patients, in certain circumstances it is acceptable. First, the request should always come from the patient. If the patient and the clinician are both religious (and especially if they are of the same religion), such a request can be met with a simple prayer. Even if their religions differ, for example, an Orthodox Jewish physician might be comfortable offering a short prayer in Hebrew or a very broadly worded prayer in English for an evangelical Christian patient. Nonetheless, patients will need to respect the moral limits of what they can reasonably request of their physicians and nurses. A Buddhist physician might understandably feel offended if asked to lay hands on the patient's head and invoke the Holy Spirit. Because of the complexity of this situation, the general guideline would be that if asked to pray with a patient, clinicians follow the patient's lead and suggest that the patient say the prayer in his or her own tradition. Clinicians may also invite chaplains to lead the prayer as the clinician remains present with the patient during that prayer.

Some clinicians will be uncomfortable praying with any patients under any circumstances. Such practitioners can respectfully decline a patient's request for prayer, acknowledging the honor of being asked, but explaining their reasons for not wishing to participate (e.g., lack of religious conviction; discomfort engaging in a particular style of prayer; worry about the effect of such intimate sharing on the physician-patient relationship).

Some clinicians will be willing to pray with patients on a case-by-case basis (e.g., in the right setting, with someone of his or her own faith, after a particularly powerful experience they have shared together, in the presence of a chaplain). Again, following the patient's lead, this is most readily morally justified if the request has been initiated by the patient. Because of differences in roles, expectations, and power differentials, physicians and nurses (as opposed to chaplains) should be extremely careful about ever proposing that they might pray with a patient. This begins to border on proselytizing unless preceded by a great deal of background information strongly suggesting a patient's openness to the practice, in a relationship of profound trust and respect (generally only after a long time of getting to know each other). Further, the suggestion must be coupled with some reason to suspect that the patient is shy about asking when the clinician has made ample indirect overtures and opportunities available to the patient so that the patient could make the request or that the patient is unable to speak or ask for prayer due to medical circumstances, but the physician has prior knowledge that prayer is important for the patient clinically. Helen was a patient of mine (Puchalski) whom I treated for fifteen years. She and her daughter also attended my church. Helen frequently talked to me about her faith and how her faith helped her cope with life's challenges. Two years before she died, I told her of her diagnosis of pancreatic cancer. As she cried out her profound pain and sadness, she asked if I would pray with her. We held hands as she spoke to God, pleading for mercy and help. A few days before she died, while I was making a house call, Helen talked to me about her fears of choking to death. She asked if I knew of a way she could calm herself. Knowing how important prayer was to her, I asked her if that might help her now. Her eyes lit up. In this moment nearing the end of her life, I sensed that my praying the words of a prayer she often used would not only be appropriate but would reflect the deep care and compassion I felt for her. I said the words of Helen's prayer; she joined me in the amen and then nodded off to a gentle sleep, calmer and less agitated.

In general, however, it is not recommended that clinicians actively seek prayer with patients. In the case of Helen, her physician knew her well and had prior knowledge of the importance of prayer in her life. Her doctor was not seeking to pray with her but utilized a spiritual resource the patient had used many times in their clinical encounter. But there are some clinicians who will actively seek to pray with patients. Such clinicians should never force prayer upon patients. Health care professionals need to be careful not to take advantage of patients' vulnerabilities. For example, it is inappropriate for a surgeon, without prior patient consent, to pray aloud over a patient when that patient is on a stretcher on the way to the operating room, possibly already premedicated. Nonetheless, there should be no objection to patients and clinicians incorporating prayer into practice if this has been arranged through formal or informal advance notification, inquiry, and mutual consent.

Praying for Patients Although there is clear precedent regarding the moral concerns around the practice of clinicians praying with patients, there is less clarity regarding clinicians who might pray privately for their patients. In this regard, the sensitivity that we need to show for every individual's beliefs and culture should apply, regardless of whether we are at the bedside of that individual or not.

One might suggest that in terms of prayer offered privately, the same rules would not apply. After all, the prayer is being done away from the clinical setting and on the clinician's personal time. However, there are many that might not be comfortable with their clinician praying for them without their knowledge. This is in part resulting from the fact that the patient's beliefs might be greatly different than that of the clinician. It is true that the prayer might be for something as harmless as hoping for healing or well-being. Yet, what if the prayer is for the patient to accept Jesus as his or her savior or see the error of his or her choice to be Buddhist? Yet it seems wrong, however, even on purely consequentialist grounds, to ask clinicians to alienate themselves from their deepest self-identifying beliefs and professional motivations in the service of an artificial neutrality. On purely secular grounds, a society would seem to have good grounds for actually encouraging clinicians to be mindful of their patients' well-being even when not in their presence, regardless of whether the patient and clinician could ever agree about whether that mindfulness could be called prayer or if a third party named God were listening.

A nurse with strong religious beliefs shared that she routinely prayed that God would give her strength and guidance in caring for her patients, believing that asking for God's blessing on her as a nurse was more respectful of her patients' diverse religious and spiritual beliefs. In another case, a Muslim family in an ICU setting shared that their prayers were for strength to be given to the health care professionals who were caring for their son.

In general, clinicians should be mindful to consider when they pray for their patients, even in private, that they be respectful of their patients' diversity of beliefs and offer a prayer that respects that individual. Clinicians should remember that there is a power differential between them and their patients and so clinicians are held by a different standard. Being aware of that allows the clinician to be conscious of boundaries and hold the patient's well-being and good ahead of their own self-interest or desire. Thus, even a private prayer should be for the well-being the patient desires.

Ethical Issues

When Patients' Beliefs Conflict with Clinicians' Treatment Recommendation Clinicians have an obligation to honor, when possible, patients' beliefs and practices even if they may conflict with the clinician's clinical agenda or hospital protocol. For example, when a Jehovah's Witness refuses blood products or when Buddhists wish to extend the time in the hospital room with their deceased loved one, it is important that those values be respected. In situations where religious parents refuse medical care for their children or for the cognitively impaired adult, the legal and ethical issues become more complicated. The issue then is whether the child or cognitively impaired adult, who may be unable to make a decision for him- or herself, needs to have an impartial legal representative who can decide what is best for that patient.

The Special Case of Miracles One infrequent but particularly vexing problem occurs when on the basis of belief in miracles the patient (or family) refuses to authorize limits on treatment that, from a biomedical perspective, have been deemed futile because the patient is imminently and irreversibly dying. Mrs. Smith was a fifty-four-year-old woman who had suffered a major heart attack. After two weeks in the ICU, Mrs. Smith had a severe myocardial infarct, which resulted in multisystem organ failure. The ICU physician approached the family about "withdrawing life support" since the patient, as determined by biomedical data, was dying. The family responded, "My loved one will be healed by God; do not stop treatment." Such expressions should not be taken at face value, but neither should they be taken lightly. Sometimes such refusals may be expressions of psychological denial. Other times they may constitute expressions of deep religious faith. Understanding the difference between positive and negative religious coping and having the knowledge to judge between these states may help clinicians to sort their way through these difficult cases. While there are research instruments to measure a patient's religious coping, the precise clinical utility of "diagnosing" patients' religious coping styles is still, at present, a matter of prudential judgment and experience, in need of a broader empirical basis. However, chaplains are trained in how to differentiate positive from negative coping and therefore are excellent resources in these situations. In the case of Mrs. Smith, the children all had different views on what their mother might want. The younger children felt that she would not want to be kept alive on a machine and that if a miracle were to occur, it would occur regardless of the machines. The oldest daughter, Mary, who was also the power of attorney and decision maker, insisted on aggressive care. Even after two neurologists declared Mrs. Smith had irreversible brain damage, Mary continued to insist on a miracle. The physicians tried to reason with Mary and even suggested that if God were to perform a miracle it would happen regardless of medical intervention. Mary became angry and threatened a lawsuit.

These disputes are clearly situations in which clinicians need to humbly acknowledge the limits of their expertise. First, science does have its limits; there are cases of seemingly miraculous recoveries. Second, clinicians would benefit from working with chaplains in these cases. Sometimes patients misunderstand the medico-moral teachings of their own religions. Sometimes these cases are intertwined with suspicions based on centuries of discrimination and marginalization from the health care system. Clinicians ought never to try to reframe the patient's belief in miracles, but should defer to chaplains or the patient's own clergy to help interpret and reinterpret the patient's theological understanding of the situation.

How conversations are handled with patients and their families is important. Usually the conversations become adversarial or misunderstood because clinicians speak from a biomedical perspective and patients or families from a religious one. It is recommended that clinicians first respect the patient's beliefs and not engage in a discussion to disprove or argue those beliefs. The best strategies are to first find common ground with the patient or family and then explore whether the beliefs have other implications for patient care—for example, quality of life, rituals, desire or request for clergy, or visit from clergy. By focusing on the whole care of the patient and not just on a decision to terminate aggressive care, clinicians can make sure conversations are more compassionate.

Sometimes all that is needed is for the clinicians to appeal to their own conscientious objection to participation in care that is futile. If done respectfully, this can help patients and families understand that the decision is being made, in one sense, by the patient's own body and, in another sense, by the attending health care professionals, but not by the family. Once relieved of the burden of believing they have been asked to give permission for their loved one to die (which may be the only way they can interpret a consent conversation regarding the forgoing of life-sustaining treatments, no matter how it is framed), they get on with the work of grieving.

Eventually, one of the physicians explained to Mary that forcing aggressive care on her mother was not helping. He gave time and space for Mary to explain her beliefs and her anger. He let her talk about her guilt that she was not there at the house when her mother had the first heart attack. He also asked the chaplain to talk with Mary and the family. With the chaplains' support, the medical team was able to hear Mary's concern in a different way. The team was able to assume directions for decisions in a way that relieved Mary of feeling responsible for stopping futile care. Eventually Mary agreed to discontinue life support that the physician and the medical team recommended. Mrs. Smith died with her family, pastor, and her friends around the bedside.

2 RECOMMENDATIONS FOR IMPLEMENTING NCP GUIDELINES AND NQF PREFERRED PRACTICES

Part 1 set forth the background, research, and organizational standards in place that support the importance of spirituality in palliative care and health care in general. This section provides recommendations and implementation strategies to realize spiritual care in palliative care. Each of the parts is organized similarly, beginning with the theoretical, empirical, and philosophical background for the topic. The background is followed by sections specific to the topic, including practice principles, available tools, ethical guidelines where appropriate, and recommendations for implementing the topic in spiritual care.

Theoretical, Empirical, and Philosophical Background

Spiritual care offers a framework for health care professionals to connect with their patients; listen to their fears, dreams, and pain; collaborate with their patients as partners in their care; and provide, through the therapeutic relationship, an opportunity for healing. "Healing" is distinguished from "cure" in this context. It refers to the ability of a person to find solace, comfort, connection, meaning, and purpose in the midst of suffering, disarray, and pain. The care is rooted in spirituality through compassion, hopefulness, and the recognition that although a person's life may be limited or no longer socially productive, it remains full of possibility (O'Connor, 1988).

Spiritual care is grounded in two fundamentally important theoretical frameworks—one is the biopsychosocial-spiritual model of care (Barnum, 1996; Sulmasy, 2002) and the other is the patient-centered care model (Institute for Alternative Futures, 2004). Integral to both of these models of care is the recognition that there is more to the care of the patient than the physical. In the patient-centered model of care, there is evidence that by engaging in shared decision making, patient health outcomes are improved. Spiritual care emphasizes the importance of the relationship between two people (Puchalski, 2004). The clinician may be the professional expert in most of the encounter, but he or she is still a human being. By relating from our humanness, we can help to form deeper and more meaningful connections with our patients.

Dignity

Integral to spiritual care is the concept of honoring the dignity of each person. Chochinov (2002) and Chochinov et al. (2002) developed an empirically based dignity model for the terminally ill. This model provides caregivers with a therapeutic map, incorporating a broad range of physical, psychological, social, and existential concerns that may affect individual perceptions of dignity. While many palliative care clinicians provide empathic care, this dignity model offers a broad framework that can be used to inform dignity-conserving care. Based on a qualitative analysis of dying patients' perceptions of their sense of dignity, three major categories emerged: illness-related issues; dignity-conserving repertoire; and social dignity inventory. These categories refer to broad issues that determine how individuals experience a sense of dignity in the course of their approaching death. Each of these categories contains several carefully defined themes and subthemes that include uncertainty about one's health status and life and death anxiety. Other critically important themes include hopefulness, being able to see life as having meaning and purpose, and generativity/legacy (the comfort attained in the belief that one is able to leave behind something lasting and transcendent of death—for example, by identifying lifetime accomplishments, contributions, and connections to life [e.g., children, good work]). These spiritual themes are often seen in the clinical setting. The dignity model is one example of a spiritual care model that seeks to address these themes in patients' care (Chochinov, 2002, 2006; Chochinov et al., 2004).

Compassion

Foundational to spiritual care is the practice of compassion; in fact, compassion can be seen as spirituality in action. In 1998, the Association of American Medical Colleges (AAMC), responding to concerns by the medical professional community and patients that medical students or physicians entering practice lacked certain humanitarian skills, undertook a major educational initiative, the Medical School Objectives Project, to assist medical schools in their efforts to respond to these concerns. The report notes that "physicians must be compassionate and empathetic in caring for patients.... They must act with integrity, honesty, respect for patients' privacy and respect for the dignity of patients as persons. In all of their interactions with patients they must seek to understand the meaning of the patients' stories in the context of the patients', and family and cultural values" (AAMC, 1999, p. 4).

Many professional medical organizations recognize the importance of compassion and spirituality. The American College of Physicians, the professional organization for practicing physicians, convened an end-of-life consensus panel that also concluded that physicians should extend their care for those with serious medical illness by attentiveness to psychosocial, existential, or spiritual suffering (Lo et al., 1999). The American Medical Association (AMA) in its *Code of Medical Ethics* (2001) states, "the physician shall be dedicated to providing competent medical care with compassion and respect for human dignity and rights."

Nursing theories also emphasize the importance of care and compassion as part of patient care (Watson, 1999). An evolutionary view of the lexicon in nursing indicates that early nursing leaders considered compassion to be the essence of nursing (Rodgers & Knafl, 1993). Unfortunately, many patients believe that the current health care system is lacking in compassion (Sanghavi, 2006). La Puma (1996) found that physicians are judged by patients' perceptions of the compassion they show to the patient and that patients want to have more compassionate physicians treating them. In an effort to enhance end-of-life care in a community hospital system, a patient survey was conducted that revealed physician compassion was an important component of care (Hodges et al., 2006). It is evident from patient stories, from concepts about healing, and from the theoretical frameworks of medicine, nursing, and social work that compassion is an essential element of clinical care.

Compassion seeks to relieve suffering and is commonly accepted as part of the human experience. The term "compassion" derives from the Latin terms *pati* and *cum*, meaning "to suffer with" ("Compassion," 2008). This implies that compassion is more than an emotion requiring a response to someone in need. This definition of compassion requires us to share in the experience by putting ourselves in the place of the one who is suffering. The definition recognizes suffering as a process and not just an isolated moment of attending to a person in need. It becomes a dynamic interaction between the compassionate person and the sufferer as they search for meaning in the midst of apparent meaninglessness. This type of compassion requires one "to become weak with the weak, vulnerable with those who are vulnerable and powerless with the powerless" (McNeill et al., 2005, p. 4). This description of compassion implies more than a sentiment; rather it is a moral imperative to do works of mercy, as in the following definition:

Compassion asks us to go where it hurts, to enter into places of pain, to share in brokenness, fear, confusion, and anguish. Compassion challenges us to cry out with those in misery, to mourn with those who are lonely, to weep with those in tears. Compassion means full immersion into the condition of being human. (McNeill et al., 2005, p. 4)

Compassion is a complex process. It is not only the sincere wish to alleviate the suffering of another, but also the desire to relieve the immediate discomfort, the cause of the suffering, and the underlying reason for the suffering. The Dalai Lama et al. (1998) described compassion as a state of mind that is nonviolent, nonaggressive and causing no harm. This implies a mental attitude based on the wish for all people to be free of suffering, and a concomitant sense of commitment, responsibility, and response toward others. This becomes a more comprehensive or all-encompassing way of looking at the scope of a compassionate response to suffering. It involves an altruistic process in which caregivers are able to overcome and eliminate their own desires, so they can be fully present to the needs of others, unencumbered by judgmental or selfish feelings and personal and professional distractions. In this way compassion has many spiritual underpinnings.

Underwood (2005) conducted a series of structured interviews with Trappist monks to gain a better understanding of their experiences and choices to provide "other-centered" compassionate love on a daily basis, and the extent of their religious motivation. The working definitions to guide the research were "giving of self for the good of the other" and "other-centered love." The study aimed to find ways that people could practice compassion. Several descriptions of compassion emerged:

    To set aside one's own agenda for the sake of, to strengthen, or to give
    life to the other
    To experience, be present, to the situation of the other
    To have a mature view of reality
    To accept yourself in order to accept others
    Being aware of one's own emotions
    Really listening
    To help another become fully themselves

Underwood (2005) identified those factors that detracted from the ability of the monks to provide compassionate love. The most common were selfishness, fear, and a desire to be liked or look good in the eyes of others. Additional factors included the need for acceptance and belonging, guilt, ego, making others feel indebted, exercising power over others, and avoiding confrontation. The study supported the need for health care professionals to confront and differentiate their needs and feelings from the needs and feelings of the patient.

Several studies on physician/patient communication styles and patient outcomes provided support for an indirect relationship between physician compassion and improved patient outcomes. In a review of twenty-one studies of the quality of physician-patient communication, several patient outcomes were related to higher quality communication, including increased physical functioning, emotional health, and decreased physical symptoms and pain (Stewart, 1995). As this review of the literature illustrates, compassion is an attitude, a way of approaching the needs of others, and of helping others in their suffering. But more importantly, compassion is a spiritual practice, a way of being, a way of service to others, and an act of love.

Susan, a cardiac unit nurse, was helping prepare her patient, Maria, for a cardiac catheterization. She prided herself on her efficiency in getting patients to the cath lab on time. As she was switching cardiac leads to different monitors, she noticed a tear in the patient's eye. She stopped what she was doing and asked Maria what she needed. Maria asked for a moment of silence to calm herself because she was terrified. Susan felt an overwhelming sense of compassion for Maria and brought herself into "the moment" with her patient. She took a deep breath, let go of her need to do her tasks quickly, reminded herself that she was called to be a nurse to serve others, and focused all her attention on Maria. Maria held Susan's hand, took a few deep breaths, and calmed herself. Susan then returned to work but maintained her connection to Maria. She continued doing her tasks, but "with intentionality." She still was able to get her patient to the cath lab on time, but what she realized was that by doing her tasks with the intention of being present to the patient, her patients and she felt more whole. In that experience she saw her work as a spiritual practice—to bring compassion to all who suffer.

The research, as well as anecdotal stories about compassion, indicates the need for greater personal awareness of, knowledge of, and skill building in compassion and spirituality to be able to possess and maintain the ability to provide compassionate care. One might even consider compassionate care as a spiritual discipline (Cutshall & Miller, 2001).

Spiritual Care Models

Spiritual care models must be grounded in the fundamental need to honor the dignity of all people and to provide compassionate presence to all patients and families. Given all the professional health care organization standards to provide compassionate care and honor and respect the dignity of patients, spiritual care must be a transdisciplinary and interprofessional model of care (Puchalski et al., 2006). The Joint Commission (2008) requires that spiritual care be offered and available for all patients in hospital settings. The National Consensus Project has deemed spiritual, religious, and existential care as integral to a patient's care and treatment.

While there is much discussion about who can provide spiritual care, the NCP Guidelines (2009) state:

> The interdisciplinary team includes professionals with skill in assessment of and response to the spiritual and existential issues common to both pediatric and adult patients with life-threatening illnesses and conditions and their families. These professionals should have education and appropriate training in pastoral care and the spiritual issues evoked by patients and families faced with life-threatening illness. (p. 49)

Chaplains and other spiritual care professionals are central to the spiritual care plan. Of all the spiritual care professionals, chaplains are trained to work within the medical world. They are board-certified specifically to work in health care settings with patients in spiritual issues. These professional chaplains are conversant with the medical world, maintain appropriate professional boundaries, and not only refrain from proselytizing but are fully respectful of the religious and spiritual differences they encounter. Many chaplains are ordained clergy, but there are also lay chaplains. The board-certified chaplain, unlike health care professionals, has no agenda to explain, cure, or eliminate disease. The chaplain seeks only to engage sufferers and to assist them in reframing their perspective of suffering in the context of life's incongruities. The chaplain is trained to provide in-depth spiritual counseling and to diagnose spiritual distress. The chaplain conveys and fosters hope so that the patient can access the hope within him- or herself and the commitment that is present and available through the respectful and dignified way he or she is treated.

The work of spiritual care is done by all members of the health care team. This includes being a compassionate presence, doing a spiritual history, and integrating spirituality into the patient's treatment plan. However, in the health care setting, chaplains are the spiritual care professionals who work with other members of the team to diagnose spiritual distress, develop the treatment plan, provide spiritual counseling, and follow up on spiritual issues.

In addition to board-certified chaplains, clergy members, spiritual directors, and pastoral counselors also have been trained to work with spiritual and religious issues. These additional spiritual care professionals generally work in outpatient settings. Members of the clergy typically work with people in their own religious congregations or people of the same denomination.

Spiritual Care and After-Death Responsibilities

Any spiritual care model must also include care of the patient and family after the patient dies. In palliative care, the continuum of care includes support of the patient's family through the patient's dying and following his or her death. The spiritual and existential care offered by palliative care teams is multidimensional and consists of education and support through the dying process, attending the funeral or wake, sending a condolence card, calling the family to offer condolence and to hear their story, follow-up phone calls, sending of grief and bereavement materials, or notification regarding bereavement support groups (Otis-Green, 2006). In addition, spiritual care providers are often called upon to assist their health care colleagues following particularly traumatic deaths and in facilitating rituals that encourage reflection and self-care to minimize compassion fatigue. Care delivered in the hours or days preceding death has a significant influence on the bereavement of the family. Practices at the time of death such as including the family in care of the body, having family members bathe or dress the deceased, or performing rituals at the death become powerful memories that can provide solace and healing.

Care does not end until the palliative care team has helped the family with their grief reactions and helped those with complicated grief to get care (Ferris et al., 2003). The NCP Guidelines (2009) state the "palliative care team follows up with some of the family after the patient dies (e.g., phone calls, attending wake or funeral) in order to offer support, and to help bring closure for the family as well as the healthcare professionals" (p. 49). The World Health Organization (WHO, 2007) asserts that "ideally, palliative care services should be provided from the time of diagnosis of life-threatening illness, adapting to the increasing needs of cancer patients and their families as the disease progresses into the terminal phase. They should also provide support to families in their bereavement" (p. 2).

Although there is no consensus as to how bereavement care should be delivered, there is a growing recognition that aftercare must be addressed. For hospice programs this has been a mandated service since the Medicare benefit was established twenty-five years ago. Hospice programs are required to follow families for thirteen months after the death. Recently this was expanded by Medicare to include the acknowledgment that a dimension of bereavement is the spiritual needs of the family and loved ones. Although there is not a consensus as to the level and detail of this support, some type of support must be provided. At a minimum this usually includes regular mailings to the family and access to trained counselors for grief issues. In addition, there has been an increasing presence of bereavement professionals at team meetings, so that any complex issues can be addressed from the beginning of hospice care.

Clinicians are also encouraged to make phone calls to family members to express sympathy. Family members greatly appreciate the calls; clinicians also can use this as a way to bring closure to significant professional relationships. The calls do not take excessive time; health care systems should support time and models for aftercare and communication with bereaved family members.

Although the majority of family caregivers will benefit from education and anticipatory guidance to normalize the dying process and grief experience, only a few will need more specialized counseling (Doka, 2008). Spiritual care professionals have a responsibility to assess and attend to those at risk for complicated bereavement (McCall, 2004). The needs of individuals are highly variable, requiring spiritual care providers to attend to lifespan issues, while providing culturally and religiously sensitive bereavement care (Hooyman & Kramer, 2006). Perhaps the model that has been established in hospice can serve as an example of best practice for palliative care and health care in general. While clinicians in all settings are overwhelmed with demands on their time, very busy oncology units, intensive care units, and other settings have initiated routine follow-up after deaths in the way of sending sympathy cards signed by the staff or involving numerous staff so that no single clinician is overwhelmed with the responsibility. Some clinicians follow up with phone calls or even visits to families within the first year of bereavement. Many clinicians attend funerals or other services for their patients both to grieve their own loss and also to show support to the families.

Practice Principles

Interdisciplinary Spiritual Care

All members of the interdisciplinary team interact with patients. This interaction involves responding to and addressing all dimensions of the care of that patient, including the spiritual, religious, and existential as well as the physical and psychological. All of these elements can provide windows into that person's suffering and his or her ability to manage that suffering. Thus, spiritual discussions should always be part of the interdisciplinary team meetings. In the interdisciplinary team, the board-certified chaplain is the expert in spiritual or pastoral care. ("Pastoral care" is a term that refers to spiritual or religious care by a chaplain or clergy, or pastoral counselor. Some health care settings now equate pastoral and spiritual care as synonymous; both terms will be used here as referring to the health care professionals that are specialists in spiritual care.) Before we can propose and explore assessment models and ways to track these issues, it is essential for the team to have a basic care model from which the practice can be based. These models act as a template for how the team envisions its work, while providing a touchstone when it is unclear how to pro-

FIGURE 2   The Casita Resilience Building Model

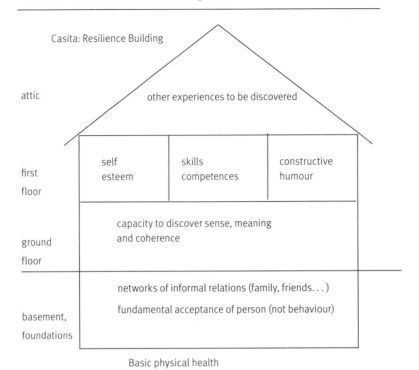

Casita: Resilience Building

attic   other experiences to be discovered

first | self | skills | constructive |
floor | esteem | competences | humour |

ground   capacity to discover sense, meaning
floor   and coherence

basement,   networks of informal relations (family, friends. . .)
foundations   fundamental acceptance of person (not behaviour)

Basic physical health

(Vanistendael, 2007)

ceed in a particular situation. A strong care model acts as the mission statement for the team so that the core ideals of the work can be maintained. The following two models and suggestions for ways to incorporate the models into spiritual care are examples.

The Casita Model   The Casita Resilience Model (see figure 2) found its roots in South America (Vanistendael, 2007). This model grew out of work being done in Chile regarding the development of resilience. It uses the image of a house to demonstrate the essentials needed in order for resilience to manifest itself in a person, family, team, or community. The model advocates a balance between the management of difficult and negative events and the ability to manifest positive attitudes and perspectives. It would seem that a model such as this would be supportive of the work of the palliative care team members, not only in how they view a patient and family, but how they view each other. This model takes the practice of palliative care out of the problem-fixing mentality generally found in medical care into a frame of mind of possibilities. Watson et al. (1999) discovered that fostering realistic hope was among the principles of spiritual care in the palliative care sector. As can be seen in the model, this hope is supported by the fact that the house is an open system where there is room for discovery.

A compelling aspect of this particular model is that at the foundation of the house is the fundamental acceptance of the person, not the person's behavior. Our work as palliative care professionals is to witness and support people as they face profound situations. It is these situations that can cause a range of behaviors or at least magnify patterns that might have been in place all their lives. So often our attitudes get mired in these behaviors and we forget that there is a person suffering underneath. Sam struggles daily with severe anxiety and paranoia, only made worse by his advanced COPD. His wife, Ann, is having a hard time dealing with his illness. She acts out at all doctors' visits. The nurses and doctors in the clinic can easily get caught up in the drama of Sam and Ann's lives. Yet underneath the drama are two individuals in deep pain and suffering. The challenge for clinicians is to not allow the drama to distract them from being present to the suffering of their patients. Hospice professionals often describe experiences of entering homes of patients and encountering familial behaviors such as a spouse's heavy alcohol use, or awareness that a husband is involved in an extramarital affair even as his wife is dying, or other behaviors such as Ann's, which may be in sharp contrast to their own values. It is important that health care providers distinguish their values and beliefs and not let those beliefs interfere with providing good care but at the same time honor their own values and not participate in a plan or action if that violates their own ethical standards. In the case of a husband having an affair, the provider can listen to all sides of a situation and offer counseling, but the ultimate action and decisions are in the hands of the patient and family. If a provider feels that the home situation is too difficult for that provider in terms of safety or values, then the provider can tell the family that perhaps another provider would be better suited and refer them to another provider. A care model such as the house reminds us to come back to that basic acceptance and openness of the situation while at the same time honoring our own values and beliefs. Approaching the patient/situation from the model can nurture a type of best practice that incorporates the holistic view proposed throughout this document.

Patient/Family-Centered Spiritual and Contemplative Practice Model   A second model that we offer for consideration adapts the known Patient/Family-Centered Spiritual and Contemplative Model of care and adds an additional layer. A basic attitude or commitment overlays the practice of the transdisciplinary team. It is also important to stress that although the patient and family are in the center, it does not mean that the interaction is one way. An exchange and dialogue are always present, whether we recognize it or not. In this way the practice of palliative care is held always in a sensibility that transcends the limitations of particular disciplines or situations. (See figure 3.)

In this model the patient and family interact with all members of the interdisciplinary team. The approach would be reflected in the team meeting, wherein different clinicians lead the discussion depending on their level of interaction with the patient and family. For example, a chaplain may note that a patient has physical pain, but the nurse or physician will make the recommendations on the treatment of the physical pain, with others on the team contributing to overall evaluation of the total pain experience. The physician may identify spiritual distress, but the chaplain will be the expert on the team who provides direction on how to treat that spiritual distress. The psychologist might diagnose demoralization and depression in addition to providing counseling to the patient. In addition to appropriate medication management, the psychologist would also defer to the chaplain to work further with the patient on meaning and purpose.

The above example describes the self-directed work team approach to patient care, in which the team works collaboratively and with a less hierarchical attitude than one often sees in transdisciplinary team functioning. Here there is an acknowledgment of roles as well as a sharing of expertise and trust in the combined efforts of the team: the whole is more than the sum of its parts. A result of this type of interac-

FIGURE 3 Spiritual and Contemplative Practice Model

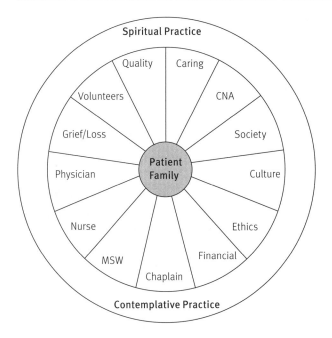

tion is that care planning can become reflective of the true needs of the patient and family. The team is then striving for the kind of comprehensive quality care that is needed for best practice to occur. This is not to say that this level of functioning is easy to achieve, but it demonstrates where we need to be setting the bar.

Within this model it is important to recognize that each health care professional has his or her own area of expertise. With regard to spiritual care, the board-certified chaplain actively and clearly collaborates with the organization's interdisciplinary patient care delivery team and should have a thorough knowledge of the services represented on the transdisciplinary team. During spiritual care delivery, the chaplain will be alert to potential patient referral opportunities. The chaplain should participate as fully as possible in the organization's transdisciplinary team meetings and work collaboratively to implement the team's care plan.

As in the case of Frank, the patient described earlier who was dying of pancreatic cancer, all members of the interdisciplinary team participated in uncovering the spiritual issue and working with the patient to help him find peace. The board-certified chaplain on the team was essential in helping guide the team regarding the spiritual interventions and working with the patient on spiritual counseling for his spiritual distress. The chaplain also communicated regularly with the team to advise how each health care provider might help the patient find self-forgiveness, as well as peace. The chaplain also connected with the patient's faith community to facilitate a reconnection.

Professional Development: Spiritual and Reflective Preparation

Clinicians are encouraged to view their relationship with the patient as a partnership where decisions are made together and where the clinician supports the patient with a philosophy that "we will get through this together." To have shared decision making, clinicians must know the values and beliefs of the patient. Finally, involvement of a larger community of caregivers is recognized as essential in the patient-centered care model. In this sense, the transdisciplinary team becomes one community, but there are other communities such as faith-based communities, families, or other communities of individuals that participate in the care of patients. Spiritual care professionals in the community include spiritual directors, pastoral counselors, faith community nurses, and clergy. Hospices also become such communities for many dying patients.

For some health care professionals, spiritual care may be intuitive but most will need to develop the knowledge and skills for providing high-quality and competent spiritual care. The ability to listen, be a compassionate presence, convey dignity, and attend to the spiritual care needs of patients and families requires awareness and growth in one's own spiritual journey. Health care professionals need to have opportunities to connect with their call to service and to understand spirituality or transcendence in their own lives. Health care providers need to have reflective preparation as part of their professional development to identify their own sense of meaning and purpose and develop as authentic whole persons. Finally, they need to have the awareness to allow themselves to be transformed by their healing experiences with their patients. A relationship and regular conversa-

FIGURE 4   Spiritually Prepared Health Care Provider

Personal Attributes

Compassion

Self-awareness

Ability to reflect on meaning of their work and contributions

Appropriate integration of personal spirituality into professional life

Open to personal transformation

Professional Skills

Training in spiritual care and compassionate presence

Competence reflective of professional discipline

Team skills and integration of multiple disciplines

Spiritual practice that supports professional work

tions with confidential and supportive persons can facilitate one's own reflection, spiritual growth, and spiritual renewal. This professional reflective developmental process allows caregivers to have the capacity for compassionate action with their patients and their colleagues.

One of my (Puchalski) medical residents, a practicing Hindu, found her spirituality affected once she started her residency program. She said that she was "spiritual from 6 p.m. to 6 a.m.," but once she came to work she felt she focused so much on the stress of the daily activity that she had not integrated her spirituality into her work. Having her residency director affirm the importance of reflective practices and attention to the spiritual dimension in the care provided by residents allowed her to share her beliefs with her colleagues and to feel safe to share her calling to serve as part of her spiritual beliefs and values.

Spiritual care also involves practicing the same values with colleagues as with patients. Thus, clinicians treat each other with respect, dignity, and compassion. Part of the preparation of the clinician is development and expression of personal attributes as well as professional skills of competence, training, contributing to an integral team, and working with many disciplines in an effective and respectful manner. Figure 4 illustrates the attributes and skills of the spiritually prepared health care provider.

Spiritual Care Framework

In studies of hospitals that have integrated spiritual interventions based on a model of compassionate care, caregivers were more able to provide the compassionate care that they aspired to (Puchalski & McSkimming, 2006). A framework of care takes into account several dimensions of spirituality, including the health care professional's sense of transcendence, meaning, purpose, call to service, connectedness to others, and transformation. In addition, the framework should address compassion as a spiritual discipline that includes being fully present to others, viewing compassion as a moral imperative with universality for all suffering individuals, and with full knowledge and experience of the profound nature of suffering. The elements of this framework are illustrated in figure 5.

The reflective process identified in this framework is undertaken by health care professionals as part of their professional development to promote awareness of their sense of transcendence, call to service, and connection to others. It helps them build on their altruism to provide compassionate presence. The process teaches them how to be fully intentional with their patients and colleagues and leads them to an ability to be full partners with their patients through illness. Finally, it enables them to be open to the transformation that can occur in healing encounters with others.

FIGURE 5   Spiritual Care Framework

Dimensions of Spirituality	Humanitarian Skills (Joint Commission on the Accreditation of Healthcare Organizations [JCAHO])*
Call to service	Compassion
Meaning and Purpose	Empathy
Transcendence Reflective Preparation	Dignity
Connectedness	Respect
Transformation	Support
	Capacity for Action

*Essential but not sufficient to alleviate suffering w/o action

(Puchalski et al., 2009)

FIGURE 6 Inpatient Spiritual Care Implementation Model

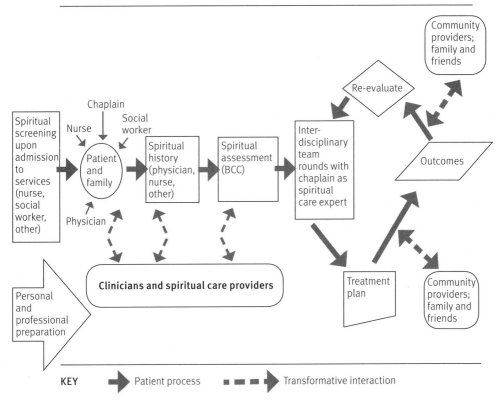

BCC: Board-certified chaplain
Clinicians: Chaplains, physicians, nurses, social workers
Community providers: Communitiy religious leaders, spiritual director, pastoral and community counselors, faith community nurses, physical therapists, occupational therapists, and others
(Puchalski et al., 2009)

In summary, a spiritual care model is a relational model in which the patient and clinicians work together in a process of discovery, collaborative dialogue, treatment, and ongoing evaluation and follow-up. Figures 6 and 7 provide two models of the ideal spiritual care model. The models are different for inpatient and outpatient settings but have similar overall goals. Clinicians may include the traditional transdisciplinary team in the hospital, long-term care, or hospice setting. But there are also community providers who may interact with the patient

FIGURE 7 Outpatient Spiritual Care Implementation Model

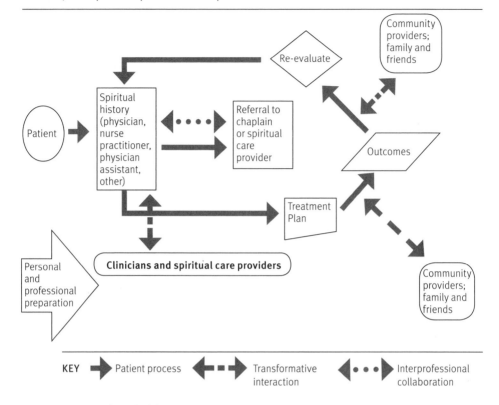

BCC: Board-certified chaplain
Clinicians: Chaplains, physicians, nurses, social workers
Community providers: Communitiy religious leaders, spiritual director, pastoral and community counselors, faith community nurses, physical therapists, occupational therapists, and others
(Puchalski et al., 2009)

and family in other settings and in the community. All parties in the spiritual care model have a potential for being transformed by the inter-action with one another. Clinicians need to do reflective work to gain insight into their own sense of spirituality, meaning, and professional call to have the capacity to provide compassionate and skillful care.

Using the inpatient model, the patient is screened initially by who-ever does the intake. These providers need to be trained in spiritual screening and to know when to refer to a chaplain for a spiritual emergency. The patient then has a spiritual history taken as part of the social history gathered for patients seeing the physician and nurse. In some settings social workers may also do the spiritual history. Depending on the spiritual concern, patients are then referred to chaplains for a complete spiritual assessment. A treatment plan is developed by the interdisciplinary team and implemented. Outcomes are measured with appropriate reevaluation and follow-up. Community clergy, religious leaders, spiritual directors, pastoral counselors, and faith community nurses may be involved in the care. Usually the coordination of community spiritual care professionals is through the chaplain.

In the outpatient setting the physician, advance practice nurse, or physician assistant do the spiritual history. These clinicians need to be connected with community resources such as chaplains who see patients in the outpatient setting, faith community nurses, spiritual directors, pastoral counselors, and religious leaders who can then be involved in outpatient referral. A similar process of reevaluation and follow-up is needed, but it falls to the physician, advanced practice nurse, or physician assistant to follow up with the spiritual caregivers in the outpatient setting.

Recommendations

1. Spiritual care should be integral to any compassionate and patient-centered health care system model of care.
2. Spiritual care models should be based on honoring the dignity of all people and on providing compassionate care.
3. Spiritual distress or religious struggle should be treated with the same intent and urgency as treatment for pain or any other medical or social problem.
4. Spirituality should be considered a patient vital sign. Just as pain is screened routinely, so should spiritual issues be a part of routine care. Institutional policies for spiritual history and screening must be integrated into intake policies and ongoing assessment of care.
5. Spiritual care models should be interdisciplinary and clinical settings should have a Clinical Pastoral Education–trained board-certified chaplain as part of the interprofessional team.

7 Spiritual History Taking and Assessment of Patients and Families

Theoretical, Empirical, and Philosophical Background

Spirituality is an essential element of health care because spirituality is, as Viktor Frankl (1963) wrote, the essence of our humanity. Spirituality speaks to what gives ultimate meaning and purpose to a person's life. It is that part of us that seeks healing and reconciliation with self or others (Foglio & Brody, 1988; Puchalski, 2002a). In this definition all people are spiritual because at some point in their life, all seek meaning and healing. Thus, spirituality, broadly defined, is inclusive of nonbelievers as well as the religious. Atheists, agnostics, spiritual but not religious, and religious patients all have an inner life that can be encompassed within the overall understanding of spirituality. There is also institutional support for the inclusion of spirituality, broadly defined, into health care. The Joint Commission (1996; 2008) requires that when a hospitalized patient requests spiritual care, it should be provided.

Spiritual Issues Facing Patients

People find many sources of meaning and purpose throughout their lives that may be transient—jobs, relationships, accomplishments, and financial success. However, the challenge for all people is to find meaning and purpose even in the midst of failed jobs, relationships, accomplishments, and unattained successes, especially at the end of life. Ultimate meaning is meaning that sustains individuals in the emptiness of their external lives, or as people face their dying. The inability to find meaning and purpose can lead to depression and anxiety. Spiritual and religious beliefs play a significant role in how people transcend their suffering to find such ultimate meaning (Wong & Fry, 1998).

Hopelessness often arises in the midst of serious illness. Studies have indicated that people who are more hopeful do better in regard to depression and other health indicators (Breitbart, 2003; Snyder et al., 1991). How people come to understand hope also varies. Initially, hope may be lodged in cure or recovery, but when that is not possible, people may have a hard time tapping into resources of hope. In those times hope may be manifested as acceptance, completing important goals or activities, living life fully in the face of difficulty, finding meaning, and eventually experiencing a good quality of life and death. Helping people restructure their thinking so that they can see hopefulness in the midst of despair is an essential part of the therapeutic process. Spiritual and religious beliefs offer a language of hope. Religious and spiritual communities offer support in the quest to find hope and meaning. (See table 3.)

Ronda was a fifty-year-old woman who had ovarian cancer. Her hope had always been for a cure. Eventually when her cancer spread and curative therapy was no longer appropriate, Ronda went into a deep depression, finding it hard to see any glimmer of hope in her desperate situation. I (Puchalski) asked Ronda to come up with a dream list for whatever time she had left. In the midst of her tears, she was able to muster up her innate sense of humor to make a joke about her remaining time. In the next few days she came up with seven things that were important to her. This gave her a sense of purpose and meaning in her life, but it also gave her hope to finish important tasks, including seeing people close to her, visiting a mountain that was a sacred place for her, making sure her parents would be taken care of, teaching a class for medical students with me, and having a party to celebrate and thank her family, friends, and caregivers for being in her life.

Religious and spiritual themes often arise in the clinical setting. People might present with a sense of meaninglessness or hopelessness. Others might present struggling with forgiveness or resentment. Illness can trigger many spiritual issues and therefore the clinical setting may be the first place where these spiritual issues arise. Religious issues can also cause distress in people's lives. For example, anger at God is common in the face of serious illness. Yet it can lead to conflict, guilt, and despair. It is important in the clinical setting to allow people to talk about that anger in a safe environment where they do not feel they will be judged. In their religious communities, patients may be told that it is wrong to be angry at God or that it reflects a weakening in one's faith to be angry at or feel abandoned by God. Yet in the clinician's office, the patient may find a safe haven to explore these feelings in greater depth. Koenig et al. (1998) found that negative religious coping was associated with poorer physical health, worse quality of life, and greater depression in medically ill hospitalized older adults, but that positive religious coping was associated with better mental health in those patients. Understanding how spirituality and religion relate to patients' understanding of their illness and their ability to cope is an important aspect of providing comprehensive patient-centered care (table 3). Spirituality may also present as a

TABLE 3 Spiritual Issues (Faced by Chronically Ill and Dying Patients)

Issue	Possible Approaches
Lack of meaning and purpose	Compassionate presence
Hopelessness	Open-ended questions
Despair	Inquiry about spiritual beliefs, values, and practices
Religious struggle	
Not being remembered	Reflective listening
Guilt/shame	Life review, listening to the patient's story
Loss of dignity	Targeted spiritual intervention
Lack of love, loneliness	Continued presence and follow-up
Anger at God/others	
Abandonment by God/others	
Feeling out of control	
Spiritual suffering	
Distress secondary to misinterpretation of religious dogma or religious or spiritual community actions that impede full development of human potential	
Trust	
Reconciliation	
Grief/loss	
Gratitude	

(Puchalski, 2002b)

TABLE 4   Sources of Spiritual Strength

Gratitude

Hope

Ability to forgive

Connection to God/transcendent/self

Support from spiritual or religious community

Peace/serenity/acceptance

Surrender

Love

Forgiveness of self

Satisfying philosophy of life

Joy

Courage

Heightened coping

Meditation

(Puchalski, Handzo, Wintz, & Bull, 2009)

source of strength for patients (see table 4). Patients often seek forgiveness, especially in end-of-life care; the ability to forgive can therefore be a strength. Connection to God or the sacred can be a positive aspect of coping for patients, as can be the ability to be grateful, find hope in the midst of suffering, and find joy in life.

Religious/spiritual struggle can be particularly challenging. Diagnosis with a life-threatening illness or other adverse life events can precipitate emotional and religious turmoil. For example, a woman in her fifties with advanced cancer told a chaplain, "Why? Why me? I just can't figure it out. And I get so depressed that I just want to give up on life altogether, you know? And I'm so very angry at God. So angry. I refuse to speak to Him. You know what I mean?" (Fitchett & Roberts, 2003, p. 25). As people attempt to integrate the reality of illness or adverse life events into their spiritual or religious beliefs, they may ask, "Why me?" or if they are religious they may ask, "God, why did you let this happen to me?" For some, this period of spiritual or religious struggle may be brief; for others it can be quite protracted.

It may lead to growth and transformation for some people and to distress and despair for others (Pargament et al., 2004). Distress may also arise from a person's misinterpretation of religious dogma or a community's harmful actions toward another that results in pain and may impede a person's full development of his or her human potential.

Since the late 1990s, evidence has accumulated about the adverse physical and emotional effects of spiritual or religious struggle. In a study of 577 hospitalized, medically ill older patients, Koenig et al. (1998) found that some aspects of religious struggle were associated with poorer physical health, worse quality of life, and greater depressive symptoms. In a two-year follow-up of this sample, Pargament et al. (2004) reported that people with chronic religious struggles had poorer quality of life, greater depression, and increased disability.

Pargament et al. (2001) also examined the effects of religious struggle on mortality of their subjects. They found that religious struggle was a significant predictor of increased mortality, even after controlling for demographic, physical health, and mental health factors. Sherman et al. (2005) found that patients with higher levels of religious struggle (i.e., negative religious coping) had greater levels of general distress and depression and higher indices of pain and fatigue, and more difficulties with daily physical functioning. Evidence from studies in other nations are consistent with these reports from the United States. Among one hundred women in Australia recently diagnosed with gynecologic cancer, higher levels of negative religious coping were associated with more depression and anxiety (Boscaglia et al., 2005). Likewise, in a sample of 156 German women with breast cancer, negative religious coping was associated with increased depression (Zwingmann et al., 2006).

Religious struggle was found to be associated with poorer quality of life and greater emotional distress among patients with diabetes and congestive heart failure (Fitchett et al., 2004), and with increased depressive symptoms among patients with end-stage congestive heart failure (Edmondson et al., 2008). Spiritual or existential struggle can also affect quality of life. Many studies have shown that people who lack meaning and purpose or lack fulfillment in their life have a poorer quality of life (Cohen et al., 1995). This growing body of evidence points to the importance of screening all palliative care patients for possible religious struggle and, where indicated, making a referral for an in-depth spiritual assessment by a professional chaplain (Boscaglia et al., 2005; Fitchett et al., 2004; Koenig et al., 1998; Pargament et al., 2001; Pargament et al., 2004; Sherman et al., 2005; Zwingmann et al., 2006).

Patients at the end of life often identify existential questions that they want to address and discuss, whether or not there are answers. These include the timeless questions about the human condition such as "Why am I here? What is the meaning of my life? Where am I going when I die? Is there a God or benevolent force in the universe? Will I be forgiven? Why do I suffer?" (Nelson-Becker, 2006). Some patients find answers to their questions, but many do not.

Nonetheless, even if specific answers are not found, patients can come to an acceptance of not having the exact answer and being with the unknown. For example, Robert was a successful physicist who lived his whole life asking questions and finding answers to those questions. He received numerous honors, including a Noble Prize for his research. But at age seventy-eight, he was diagnosed with dementia. As I (Puchalski) sat on the edge of his bed in the hospital, he cried out, "Why is this happening? My mind is all I ever had." As I sat with him, the silence being drowned out by his tears, I knew there was nothing I could say that would take away the intense pain he was feeling. And Robert knew there was no answer. We did not talk of answers. He wanted to be heard and wanted some reassurance that he would not be alone in the coming years of his progressive dementia. Over the next few months, he was able to find an inner peace with his situation. He told me at one visit, "After all these years of finding answers, I am now faced with questions that are unanswerable and to which I have to surrender."

Palliative care professionals do well to hear these difficult questions and the anguish and sorrow and, sometimes, the joy that come behind them. Patients communicate not only with words, but with their emotions in very tangible and sometimes intense ways. Practitioners need to be able to hear all of these expressions of grief, longing, and compassion. To do so means reflecting on and coming to terms with their own life questions and emotional repertoire. Spiritually sensitive palliative care practice does not condemn or seek to rationalize away patient beliefs, but rather asks questions and seeks understanding through that process. In spiritual care, asking the right questions is key. Further, from a narrative therapy standpoint, patients who share their personal perspective and stories about their views of illness and interpretation of life events can experience a form of spiritual and emotional healing. This is a healing that is hope-inducing even where hope for the body's healing itself is absent.

Creating an Environment of Trust

The first step in communicating with patients about spiritual issues is to communicate a genuine interest and compassion for the patient. In the consensus conference sponsored by the Association of American Medical Colleges (AAMC) and the George Washington Institute for Spirituality and Health, medical educators, clinicians, medical ethicists, and chaplains developed guidelines for spiritual care (Puchalski, 2006b). Of particular importance was that clinicians should create environments where patients feel they can trust their clinician and share whatever concerns they have, including spiritual concerns. By creating an atmosphere of caring and compassion and demonstrating a willingness to be open to whatever is of concern to the patient, the interaction becomes focused in a patient-centered model of care. In this model there is recognition that a patient's understanding of illness can be affected by many factors, including spiritual and religious beliefs and practices (Institute for Alternative Futures, 2004).

How can an environment of trust be created? Patients trust health care professionals who respect them and honor who they are as people, not just disease entities. They want to be heard and want to know that what they share will be respected and not judged. Karen had seen many physicians and advance practice nurses for a chronic headache. She had a history of depression, so the providers assumed her symptoms were related to her depression and anxiety. Karen told them that she felt it might be a brain tumor, but no one listened to her ideas. Eventually, she left the clinical practice, looking for another physician. Unfortunately, she had been hurt by not having providers listen to her, so she was not trusting of any "white coats," as she later told me (Puchalski). We just talked of lots of things: her symptoms, her love of animals, her family, and her beliefs. Eventually she shared her fears, including the one about having a brain tumor. No one on my team judged her as being irrational. She was taken seriously and respected. Unfortunately, tests revealed a tumor, but it was caught early enough that she had a good outcome. Trust is important and the way to build that trust comes from the recognition that the health care professional–patient encounter is first and foremost a relationship based in respect and compassion.

Spirituality Across the Life Cycle

Acknowledgment of the spiritual self plays a key role in understanding relationships throughout the life course. Thus, any model of assessment must include a developmental perspective. Spiritual growth and development is a life-long journey. Spiritual development often parallels emotional development (Kelcourse, 2004). In childhood, the main psychosocial tasks include development of trust, autonomy, and initiative. Spiritually, children start making meaning of a world that is new to them, a world that is gradually becoming part of their life.

Religion often plays a role at this time if the child's family is religious. This is a time of extrinsic religiosity, a time when children are exposed to rituals and religious customs of the family. Clinically, this might be manifested as a clear, concrete vision of what life after death may mean, for example, a picture of heaven with a grandfather-like God. In adolescence, the primary psychosocial task is identity. Spiritually, the adolescent begins to accept conventional ways of finding meaning in life but also begins to question what has been offered to him or her by parents and teachers. It is a time of movement from extrinsic to intrinsic faith. Clinically, a dying adolescent might struggle with what he or she believes but might revert back to what his or her conventional beliefs are if he or she has not determined what his or her own beliefs are.

Early adulthood is a time of establishing a career and intimate relationships. Spiritually, the young adult develops a personal faith or way of making meaning in life by reflecting on what has been handed on and determining what elements of this faith or meaning-making he or she will integrate as his or her own. This is often called a time of intrinsic faith. A young adult who has established his or her own faith will use that as a foundation for dealing with illness. But many people sacrifice attention to spiritual development in favor of intellectual and career development. So, in time of crisis, they may revert to childhood faith, sometimes called "foxhole faith."

In adulthood, generativity is the key psychosocial task, one of establishing oneself securely in one's professional and family or relational life. At this time, spirituality is expressed in the integration into oneself of much that was suppressed or unrecognized in the interest of a career or family. Some refer to this stage as holistic spirituality. It may be a deep time of searching for what is meaningful beyond the external.

Spirituality may be expressed in religious terms but also in nature, beauty, pets, people, or other beliefs. Clinically, illness may actually push an adult onto a spiritual path, especially if the illness prevents the person from working or doing the things that were meaningful. As people grow older, they often become satisfied with the achievement of career goals and find a deep sense of meaning for life in their self and the world. This is also a time of acknowledging loss and disappointments, of navigating the joys as well as the sorrows of life. Many arrive at a place of peace and understanding regarding the universal value and goodness of life and of all that constitutes one's world. The adult who goes through this part of spiritual growth comes to an acceptance of the paradoxes of life. Clinically, this journey may be intensified in illness and particularly in end-of-life care, and some patients may not arrive at this peace. One goal of care would be to provide the support and environment for people to explore these deep issues of existence and find some peace in or acceptance of their life.

Spiritual development often does not move along in a linear fashion (Fowler, 1995). Also, many times spiritual growth does not parallel professional or personal development. Illness or dying may be the triggers for deeper questioning. But if people have not had the opportunity to focus on spiritual developmental issues, they may experience spiritual distress in the context of illness and may need to revert to their childhood spirituality for support. The beliefs and practices they valued as children may not support them or help them in their time of illness and stress.

Awe is the primary spiritual attitude that children experience. But when a religious dimension is added to the child's life, it can either foster or diminish that spiritual awakening. Religion fosters this awakening if ritual and dogma support a growing awareness of the transcendent, so that the growth of awe in the life of the child is nourished and encouraged. Religion can diminish or retard spiritual development in the childhood stage if it is rule centered or emphasizes a punishment/reward approach to dealing with the transcendent (Fowler, 1995). Neglect or abuse can also dampen or destroy the child's enthusiasm for the transcendent. This can be evident again in the way people handle illness, stress, or dying. If their sense of the transcendent has been nurtured, they are likely to have positive religious coping. If, on the other hand, they have had a rule-centered approach, it is more likely they will experience negative religious coping. Pargament et al. has also demonstrated this in their work on religious coping (1998). People who have a partnership relationship with God or find support in their religious communities have better psychological coping than those who see the illness as a punishment from God.

For example, Benjamin was a sixty-year-old diagnosed with lung cancer. He had smoked all his life. He was devastated when the doctors told him of his diagnosis but also told him that he had a reasonable chance of cure with surgery and radiation. On a follow-up visit, he told the physicians that he would decline surgery. On further questioning, Benjamin said that he did not deserve treatment, as he caused the illness and this was his punishment from God. Benjamin had been raised a Christian but rarely attended church in his adult life. His perception of God was the judging God he studied about in grammar school. Working with a chaplain helped Benjamin reflect on his relationship with God as he understood God as a child and now as an adult. Eventually he was able to see God differently, talk with the pastor from his wife's church, and accept his illness as an illness that he could chose freely for which to seek therapy.

A life-course perspective expands our conception of spiritual connections because it includes a number of different factors that move beyond consideration of the individual alone (Bengtson & Schaie, 1999; Elder, 2001; Hooyman & Kiyak, 2005). This perspective includes family structure and historical and social processes as well as the socially constructed meanings that evolve through transitions and in communication patterns related to an individual. While a lifespan perspective looks at antecedents and consequences of behavior across two or more life stages, the life-course perspective includes consideration of the environment in which a particular life is lived. Time, historical and social contexts, and personal choices are the major themes that a life-course perspective includes in working with individuals.

Time is an important factor in several ways. The timing of family transitions can be a source of spiritual pain/struggle or spiritual strength. For example, individuals whose grandparents die when they are young may experience the loss of the grandparents as abandonment, while those who experience a lifelong relationship with their grandparents and are able to witness the birth of their own grandchildren may experience that birth as spiritual grace. Furthermore, the larger societal historical narratives also intertwine with individual spiritual histories. Working through financial difficulties in the Great Depression of the 1930s or losing a child as a casualty of war in the mid- to late twentieth and early twenty-first centuries are to some extent shared communal experiences. While the impact is personal and individual, others in society can offer support and hope as the patient struggles to find meaning at the time of the event or through the consequential effects that come later (e.g., as a parent lives the reminder of his or her lives without the companionship of that child).

Patients are also affected by the social contexts of their lives. Ageism, racism, and sexism can cause individuals to feel marginalized, suppress the spiritual self, and make unexpected adjustments while coping with their lives. Patients interact with the social context of their environment and are in turn touched in reciprocal fashion. For some individuals, societal oppression leads to remarkable individual resilience and a strengthening of formal communal religious institutions, as has occurred in the African American community. Societal structures also change. Many religious denominations have encountered theological changes, such as changes in ritual after the Second Vatican Council in Catholicism and entrance of women into formal priesthood roles in some mainline Christian and Jewish faiths. For patients who are closely affiliated with a religious denomination, these changes can affect personal views and approval to consider new forms of spiritual and religious expression. There is an interchange on a micro and macro level as patients are affected by larger discourses and in turn affect or influence them. Knowledge about these influences or being open to learning about them from patients can facilitate development of a therapeutic relationship and communication about spiritual matters.

The life course is also shaped by decisions and actions a person chooses that affect later life events. Individual life events such as spiritual highs and lows, peak and nadir experiences help shape a patient's worldview. The personal timing of events such as age of marriage or of retirement also gives meaning to life and to the embedded nature of family relationships. A wider array of family structures including same-sex partnerships, multiethnic marriages, and multigenerational families make room for a concomitantly wider array of spiritual and religious spectrums within a single family grouping. These differences in life situation and beliefs and values can make communication quite complex. Transitions (birth, marriage, death) are viewed as sacred, but the spiritual rituals intended to facilitate celebration or comfort may not be perceived the same way by all family members. It is important to offer the space for sacred rituals in a way that is helpful to the patient, however, and help the family find ways to honor those transitions in the midst of what is happening to the patient.

There is an inherent richness and complexity to human lives. When one acknowledges the vertical influences of time as well as the social influences on spiritual development, and when one recognizes that spirituality itself is an ongoing process in people's lives, the helping professional is able to relate to patients in a respectful way that opens discussion rather than closes it. The conversations that emerge can center on any area important to the patient when trust in the relationship has been established. This holistic approach can be a further aid to healing.

Spirituality as an Element of Cultural Awareness

Spiritual assessment must also take into consideration how the complex and multidimensional phenomenon of culture influences the delivery of quality palliative care (Otis-Green, 2007). The impact of culture is magnified during times of crisis. It matters more to participate in important cultural rituals when one is feeling vulnerable, suffering, or in pain (Otis-Green et al., 2002). Culture influences how we cope with challenges and can provide structure to an otherwise untenable situation. The biopsychosocial-spiritual perspective of care (Sulmasy, 2002) coupled with the National Consensus Project Guidelines for Quality Palliative Care (NCP, 2009) remind us that a consideration of a patient and family's culture and life stage is necessary if we are to holistically address suffering.

Knowledge about cultural difference provides a second lens that assists in building deep-level relationships with clients to facilitate spiritual discussions. Psychologists have identified a principle referred to as correspondence bias (Epley et al., 2002; Gilbert & Malone, 1995). This bias may lead one to ascribe a particular personality trait or dispositional explanation for behavior when, in fact, the behavior may reflect cultural differences. Patients from Asian cultures tend to have a more collectivist frame of action for behavior and value in-group harmony and balance (Yang, 1995). For example, they may not want to make advance directive decisions without consulting family members first, or may even ask family members to decide for them (Ko, 2008). Thus, explanations from Eastern viewpoints for behavior are determined more by the situation than the individual. In Western cultures, the emphasis tends to remain on individual decisions and autonomy. Spirituality, too, may be viewed as a collective expression or a personal one.

With increasing levels of immigration in the United States, some patients come from contexts where multiple cultural/spiritual beliefs coexist. For instance, in China and Japan, Buddhist and Christian practices may coincide with Taoist beliefs and ancestor worship or Confucianism and Shintoism. These multiple spiritual and religious contexts are respected and honored within a single family in ways that may be puzzling to a palliative care professional. Inclusion of culturally based or community-based healers who can reinforce palliative care goals and may even assist patients and families in strengthening positive communication can be an asset. Overall, it is important to consider how spiritual beliefs are expressed within a unique culture and may be used as a mechanism to transform suffering (Chow & Nelson-Becker, in press).

What we pay attention to is determined by how we perceive the world (Markus & Kitayama, 1991; Nisbett & Masuda, 2003). Much information may be processed differently by people from different cultures.

There are also culturally based healers who are traditionally sought out by patients for healing rituals and practices. While not necessarily members of the typical spiritual care professions and not licensed within the U.S. medical system, these healers may provide important comfort and resources for patients and families. It would be important for health care providers to be aware of such individuals and integrate them if possible into the care plan.

Cultural and spiritual competence should include familiarity with ways patients connect to formal religious institutions and the role of informal spiritual beliefs on health behavior (Congress, 2004). To respect patients of differing cultural and spiritual backgrounds, the practitioner must pay attention to his or her own intuition and reasoning about the best ways to interact with the patient and the situation, sorting out the origins of his or her own beliefs and being willing to step away from his or her own cultural or spiritual reference points. Questioning his or her own assumptions about the patient's expression or lack of expression of spiritual needs will increase the opportunity for spiritual connections and growth for both patient and practitioner.

Practice Principles

Addressing Spiritual Issues in the Clinical Setting:
The Initial Spiritual Encounter

How patients and families come to share their spiritual story is the crux of the assessment. Ethical issues in spiritual care begin when one is deciding how and when to elicit patients' needs and preferences for spiritual care. Ample anecdotal evidence supports the notion that having patients check a box about whether they would like to see a chaplain is an extremely limited screening tool for assessing spiritual needs. The motivation for using such a question as a screening tool are that it is relatively simple, routine, and unlikely to be offend anyone. However, significant numbers of patients with important spiritual needs who could be helped by chaplains or other members of the health care team are missed when this is all that is done. Some patients are too sick and just check "no" to everything. If they cannot answer easily, the default reply is generally "no." Patients may not be imminently close to death and harbor the false notion that chaplains ought not be called until the last moment, or patients may be of a minority religion or not religious and believe spiritual care could not meet their needs. If, as we argue, attending to patients' spiritual needs is a moral mandate, it would seem that there is a compelling moral case to be made for doing a better job of eliciting patients' needs and preferences regarding spiritual care.

One way to increase the likelihood of reaching those in need might be to have routine visits of all hospitalized patients by a board-certified chaplain or other equivalently prepared spiritual care professional. This seems preferable to the alternative of limiting spiritual care visits only to patients who have requested them or those being seen by palliative care or enrolling in hospice. One important reason to cast the net widely is that the presenting issue that leads to a palliative care consults or hospice enrollment could just as easily be a spiritual issue as a biomedical issue like pain or nausea. Spiritual care professionals are skilled in identifying these spiritual issues.

A counterargument to making spiritual care visits and assessments routine for all patients would be that this might be offensive to some patients who have no religious affiliation or do not share the religion of the chaplain. However, contemporary chaplaincy care approaches patients in an open interfaith manner, and chaplains who have been specifically trained in hospital-based spiritual care are skilled in eliciting and addressing the spiritual needs of religious and nonreligious patients alike, recognizing that spiritual issues may include but transcend religious specific issues. By adhering to the rule of following the patient's lead, a conscientious chaplain who opens the patient's door unannounced will also know how to respect a patient's request to close that door and leave.

Another objection might concern the optimal use of resources. This objection can be decisive in some cases. Routine visits by chaplains are feasible only in institutions that have well-staffed pastoral or spiritual care departments. An institution with a low ratio of chaplains to patients might have to rely on other screening methods, such as spiritual histories by nurses, to trigger chaplain visits to patients. Nonetheless, such an institution's low ratio of chaplains to patients could be legitimately critiqued as an ethical problem, using arguments outlined elsewhere in this book.

Is it acceptable to challenge a patient who declines spiritual care?

Some might think that the principle of respect for patients implies that one not make repeat visits to those who have declined spiritual care. Prudence suggests, however, that one not rule out the possibility that respect might, in particular circumstances, demand the opposite. Chaplains often tell an anecdote about a patient who angrily kicked the chaplain out on the first, second, third, fourth, and fifth visits, only to welcome him into her room on the sixth visit with the words, "Well, I guess you really do care about me." Consider the fact that a physician can, under the proper circumstances, probe the reasons for a patient's refusal of a medical test or treatment to be sure that the patient's decision is based upon a correct understanding and truly reflects that patient's most fundamental self-identifying moral and personal commitments. Such probing, if done with care and concern, shows the greatest possible respect for the patient. Likewise, a patient's refusal of spiritual care might not seem, from the perspective of the care team, to be in the patient's best interests. Such a refusal might require some gentle probing to be sure that the refusal is well thought out and based upon correct information. In some cases, such as that described in the previous anecdote, the refusal may actually be a way of communicating an indirect message: a way of asking whether anyone cares enough to keep coming back.

It is therefore sometimes a mistake to take a refusal of spiritual care at face value. Clinicians need to use the same communication skills as they use for other issues they probe. For example, they might say, "You continue to be in a lot of pain; we have addressed the physical and emotional aspects and you still have pain. You have also said that you feel despair and a sense of meaninglessness. These are spiritual and existential issues. I feel strongly that a chaplain could help you a lot. It might also help with your overall pain." One respectful way to approach this might be for the clinician to approach the patient to say that other patients have often reported that they initially did not want a chaplain visit, but that as time passed on, things changed—they did in fact want to see a chaplain. In the end patients can refuse any clinicians' recommendations, but it is the obligation of clinicians to communicate their clinical decisions to the patients in order to give the patients as much information as possible in order for that patient to make a truly informed decision.

Thus, the first step in spiritual care is to ensure that all patients have a chaplain visit. But are chaplains the only professionals that can address spiritual issues? Who is responsible for eliciting the spiritual needs of patients at the end of life and assuring that proper spiritual care is rendered? In the team care approach we advocate, this responsibility belongs, in part, to all members of the team, even though the greatest responsibility for delivering these services might fall to the chaplain. Nurses, for instance, may do spiritual histories at the time of admission to a hospital or hospice program and make appropriate referrals. Physicians may discover patients' spiritual needs in the course of routine intake assessment. While the chief responsibility for conducting more extensive spiritual assessments and spiritual or pastoral care might belong properly to the chaplain, all health care providers bear some responsibility.

Do Patients Want Clinicians to Address Their Spiritual Concerns?

Patients do want spiritual care from physicians and other health care professionals. Initial research suggests that between 41 and 94 percent of patients want their physicians to address spiritual issues. In one survey, even half of the nonreligious patients thought physicians should inquire politely about patients' spiritual needs (Ehman et al., 1999). This is particularly true if patients are at the end of life or diagnosed with a serious illness. In numerous surveys, patients indicate their preference to have a more integrated approach to their care with their spiritual issues addressed by their health care professionals. Ehman et al. (1999) found that 85 percent of patients noted that their trust in their physician increased if that physician addressed their spiritual concerns, 95 percent of the patients who reported that spirituality was important wanted their doctor to be sensitive to their spiritual needs and to integrate it in their treatment, and 50 percent of the patients for whom spirituality was not important felt that physicians should address spiritual issues in the case of serious and chronic illness. McCord et al. (2004) reported that patients in a family practice setting felt it was important for physicians and health care providers to address their spiritual issues and beliefs. In this study, 95 percent of patients wanted their spiritual beliefs addressed in the case of serious illness, 86 percent when admitted to a hospital, and 60 percent during a routine history. These results are also corroborated by surveys regarding patients' desire for nursing attention to their spiritual concerns. The authors of this text (Puchalski and Ferrell) and their colleagues also recently concluded a study using the FICA spiritual assessment tool with seventy-six oncology patients. Findings of that study also demonstrated that patients value having spiritual needs assessed and that routine assessment facilitates referrals for spiritual care (Borneman et al., in press)

Physicians have generally been reluctant to address patients' spiritual concerns in practice. In one study, oncologists rated the importance of spiritual distress low compared with other clinical concerns they felt they were responsible for addressing (Silvestri et al., 2003). In addition, studies have shown that health care professionals fail to address the spiritual needs of patients with "Do Not Resuscitate" (DNR) orders. Physicians make referrals to chaplains or otherwise address the spiritual needs of patients with DNR orders less than 1 percent of the time (Sulmasy et al., 1992).

Some of the reasons for resistance to addressing spirituality in the clinical setting include lack of time, concern that it opens the door to inappropriate behavior such as proselytizing, and not having a clear definition of spirituality (Sloan et al., 2000). Anther reason is the clinicians' fear that they will do more harm or trigger an existential crisis for the patient and then not have the resources to help them. Clinicians may resort to clichés as a way of protecting themselves or because they do not know what else to say. This underscores the importance of working with chaplains and other spiritual care professionals. In this section we provide some brief spiritual history tools that can be used in the clinical setting. Ethical guidelines and boundaries that address some of the above-mentioned concerns are discussed in the ethics and boundaries sections in chapters 4, 5 and 9.

Communication about Spiritual Issues

Communication with patients and families about spiritual issues ranges from identification of spiritual issues to formal assessment (Lo et al., 2002; Puchalski & Romer, 2000). Thus, there are four basic ways to approach communication about spiritual issues:

1. Recognize spiritual themes, spiritual distress, or suffering.
2. Respond to patient's statements about spiritual, religious, or existential issues.
3. Explore patient's spiritual expressions or symbols such as religious jewelry, inspirational books at bedside, religious clothing, or verbal outcry to God or higher power.
4. Conduct a formal spiritual history, screening, or assessment.

The first three approaches can be done by anyone on the care team. During the clinical encounter, one should listen for expressions of these themes and follow up. For example, a patient may allude to a sense of meaninglessness. The professional may identify this as an expression of demoralization and elicit more conversation to identify appropriate treatment options. Patients may express spiritual or existential issues, for example, in asking, "Why is this happening to me?" It is important to respond to these types of questions with statements that invite open-ended responses (e.g., tell me more) or acknowledge the patient's struggles (e.g., I hear that this is a hard time for you and that you are trying to make sense of this situation). By trying to answer these often unanswerable questions, the clinician could miss the opportunity to hear the patient's existential distress. Providing answers would close off the opportunity for space that allows the patient to share whatever is of concern to him or her.

Patients may also voice explicit spiritual or religious beliefs. For example, a patient may make references to God or a higher power, or may mention helpful practices such as meditation or yoga. Or a patient may cry out, "God, why are you doing this to me?" The clinician can follow up by asking more about these practices or spiritual expressions. Clinicians do not need to be experts in all spiritual or religious beliefs and practices; they can learn from their patients about what is important to them.

One can also simply observe what the patient is wearing or what types of resources are at the bedside. Patients may wear religious or spiritual jewelry, or have religious or spiritual reading material at their bedside. Clinicians can acknowledge these objects and ask questions in reference to what the patient is wearing or reading—for example, to ask if the rosary has a special significance or to share how they first came to own a prayer book. This could open up the conversation to the meaning of these symbols or articles to the patient.

Listening Skills

A spiritual history involves more than simply asking questions. First, it is important to create an environment of trust so the patient knows that what he or she shares will be respected. Second, it is critical to be open to listening to the patient's story, not just the medical facts. Hence, when someone shares about meaning and purpose or despair, these issues need to be attended to with compassionate presence and full attention. The clinician should listen to the content of what is said, the emotion and manner in which it is said, and the spiritual meanings. Together the patient and the one who listens form the landscape of memory and the context for the present act of meaning-making (Nelson-Becker, 2008). Anecdotally, medical students have often said that "something in the room changes when I ask patients the spiritual history." Both patient and clinician may sense when this space has opened up and entrance has been gained into what some call a sacred or healing space. Being fully present can open a healing space that acknowledges faith-based or spiritual practices (Milstein, 2008). Asking a spiritual history can also open up a space where the patient can feel increased trust in his or her health care professional. (McCord et al., 2004).

Spiritual Screening, History, Assessment

A spiritual screening, history, and assessment are more formal parts of the medical history during which the patient or family is asked about their spiritual or religious beliefs. In general, nonchaplain clinicians do a spiritual screening or history and chaplains do the spiritual assessment. When each of these inquiries occurs depends on the setting and who is asking the question. In hospitals, nursing homes, or hospices, the spiritual screening is done by the nurse or social worker upon triage or admission. The purpose is to assess for spiritual emergencies that may require a chaplain immediately. Once the initial admission process is completed, then a spiritual history is taken as part of the intake or complete history after the initial triage. In outpatient settings, the spiritual screening might not occur. If the patient comes to the physician's office and is in distress, a spiritual screening might be done as part of the initial conversation with the physician, advanced practice nurse, or physician assistant. Screening for spiritual distress might also occur in the context of the spiritual history.

Spiritual Screening Spiritual screening or triage is a quick determination of whether a person is experiencing a serious spiritual crisis and therefore needs an immediate referral to a board-certified chaplain. Spiritual screening helps identify which patients may benefit from an in-depth spiritual assessment. Like screening in other disciplines, spiritual screening is designed to provide initial information about whether a patient may be experiencing a high level of religious or spiritual distress or a possible spiritual crisis. A growing body of research suggests that religious and spiritual struggles are associated with poorer quality of life and poorer psychological adjustment for cancer patients and others (Boscaglia et al., 2005; Fitchett et al., 2004; Koenig et al., 1998; Pargament et al., 2001; Pargament et al., 2004; Sherman et al., 2005; Zwingmann et al., 2006).

In her work on spiritual care, Taylor (2003) recommends a two-stage process of screening followed by in-depth assessment for nurses. Good models of religious or spiritual screening employ a few simple questions that can be asked by any health care professional in the course of more general screening. Examples of questions could be "How important is religion and spirituality in your coping?" and "How well are those resources working for you at this time?" (Fitchett & Risk, 2009).

Spiritual History Spiritual history-taking is the process of interviewing a patient and asking his or her questions about his or her life to come to a better understanding of the patient's spiritual needs and resources. Compared to screening, history-taking employs a broader set of questions to capture salient information about needs, hopes, and resources to identify spiritual, religious, or existential distress. The history questions are usually asked in the context of a comprehensive examination by a clinician who is primarily responsible for providing direct care or referrals to specialists such as professional chaplains. Information from the history permits the clinician to understand how spiritual concerns could either complement or complicate the patient's overall care. It also allows the clinician to incorporate spiritual care into the patient's overall care plan. Unlike spiritual screening, which requires limited training, those doing a spiritual history should have some training in and comfort with these issues and how to engage patients in this discussion.

Spiritual Assessment   Spiritual assessment refers to an extensive, in-depth, ongoing process of actively listening to a patient's story as it unfolds in a relationship with a professional chaplain and summarizing the needs and resources that emerge. The summary includes a spiritual care plan with expected outcomes that should be communicated to the rest of the treatment team. Unlike history-taking, the major models for assessment are not built on a set of questions that can be employed in an interview. Rather, the models are interpretive frameworks that are applied based on listening to the patient's story as it unfolds in the clinical relationship. Because of the complex nature of these assessments and the special clinical training necessary to engage in them, they should be done only by board-certified chaplains. The assessment may be done under some circumstances by other health care professionals who have had extensive training and clinical pastoral education.

An early and influential model for religious/spiritual assessment was developed by psychologist Paul Pruyser (1976). In his model, which was addressed to parish clergy, chaplains, and pastoral counselors, Pruyser suggested they attend to seven aspects of a person's religious life. See table 5.

Another model for assessment is the 7 x 7 model, developed by Fitchett (2002). The 7 x 7 model employs a functional and multidimensional approach to spiritual assessment. As seen in table 6 below, the 7 x 7 model has two broad divisions: a holistic assessment and a multidimensional spiritual assessment.

In *The Discipline for Pastoral Care Giving*, Art Lucas (2001) describes an assessment model focused on the patient's concept of the holy, meaning, hope, and community. It explicitly places the work of spiritual assessment in the context of the clinical process and its cycle of assessment, care plan, intervention, and reassessment, which aligns it with the models used by physicians and nurses. All of these

TABLE 5   Guidelines for Pastoral Diagnosis

1. **Awareness of the Holy**

    What, if anything, is sacred, revered?

    Any experiences of awe or bliss, when, in what situations?

    Any sense of mystery, of anything transcendent?

    Any sense of creatureliness, humility, awareness of own limitations?

    Any idolatry, reverence displaced to improper symbols?

2. **Providence**

    What is God's intention toward me?

    What has God promised me?

    Belief in cosmic benevolence

    Related to capacity for trust

    Extent of hoping vs. wishing

3. **Faith**

    Affirming vs. negating stance in life

    Able to commit self, to engage

    Open to world or constricted

4. **Grace or Gratefulness**

    Kindness, generosity, the beauty of giving and receiving

    No felt need for grace or gratefulness

    Forced gratitude under any circumstances

    Desire for vs. resistance to blessing

5. **Repentance**

    The process of change from crookedness to rectitude

    A sense of agency in one's own problems or one's response to them vs. being a victim vs. being too sorry for debatable sins

    Feelings of contrition, remorse, regret

    Willingness to do penance

6. **Communion**

    Feelings of kinship with the whole chain of being

    Feeling embedded or estranged, united or separated in the world, in relation with one's faith group, one's church

7. **Sense of Vocation**

    Willingness to be a cheerful participant in creation

    Signs of zest, vigor, liveliness, dedication

    Aligned with divine benevolence or malevolence

    Humorous and inventive involvement in life vs. grim and dogmatic

(Pruyser, 1976)

TABLE 6   The 7 x 7 Model for Religious/Spiritual Assessment

Holistic Assessment	Spiritual Assessment
Medical Dimension	Belief and Meaning
Psychological Dimension	Vocation and Obligations
Family Systems Dimension	Experience and Emotions
Psychosocial Dimension	Courage and Growth
Ethnic, Racial, or Cultural Dimension	Ritual and Practice
Social Issues Dimension	Community
Spiritual Dimension	Authority and Guidance

(Fitchett, 2002)

models are indicated for use with patients from many different religious or spiritual traditions and belief systems.

Spiritual Screening and History Tools

Spiritual Screening   A patient entering the hospital, hospice, or a long-term setting is usually interviewed by an admissions clerk, nurse, or social worker. The person doing the intake can ask: "Is spirituality or religion important to you? Are those resources helping you now?" If the person answers yes to the first question and no to the second, that should generate an automatic chaplain referral. If the person answers yes to both or no to both, then no chaplain referral may be needed at this time, although a patient reporting spirituality to be important and currently helping may often request chaplaincy referral at this time of life transition. The patient then moves through admission to fuller clinical interviews with physicians or nurses and at that time the spiritual history can be taken and the algorithm developed by Fitchett and Risk (2009) can be used to support this decision making.

Spiritual History   Health care professionals use clinical history tools to collect and document clinical information. The spiritual history can

FIGURE 8   Religious Struggle Screening Protocol

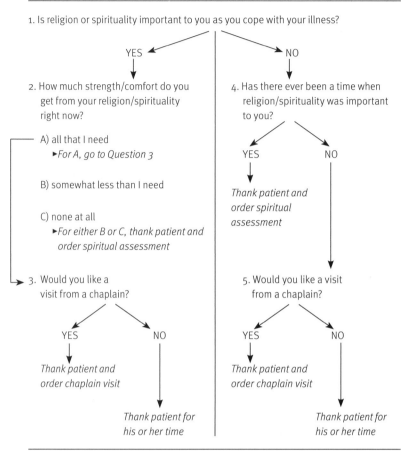

1. Is religion or spirituality important to you as you cope with your illness?

YES ← → NO

2. How much strength/comfort do you get from your religion/spirituality right now?

A) all that I need
▶For A, go to Question 3

B) somewhat less than I need

C) none at all
▶For either B or C, thank patient and order spiritual assessment

3. Would you like a visit from a chaplain?

YES   NO

Thank patient and order chaplain visit

Thank patient for his or her time

4. Has there ever been a time when religion/spirituality was important to you?

YES   NO

Thank patient and order spiritual assessment

5. Would you like a visit from a chaplain?

YES   NO

Thank patient and order chaplain visit

Thank patient for his or her time

(Fitchett & Risk, 2009)

be integrated into these tools. For example, the spiritual history has been integrated into the social history section of the clinical database in many settings. (See figure 9.) A spiritual history is as important as any other part of the clinical history. When conducting a clinical history, clinicians target specific areas. Simply listening to themes alone will not elicit all the information needed to provide good medical care. Thus, specific questions need to be asked to target areas of information regarding life events such as depression, social support, domestic violence, and sexual preferences and practices. Patients may not

FIGURE 9   Social History Section of an Initial Interview

Important relationships; sexual history

Occupational history

Avocation interests

Smoking, alcohol/drugs, seat belts, domestic violence, mood concerns

Wellness/prevention: exercise, nutrition, spiritual, religious, or existential beliefs, practices, and values

(Puchalski & Blatt, 2000)

volunteer information to a clinician unless they are invited to share in sensitive areas. This is particularly true of spirituality. While patients are interested in having spirituality integrated into their care, it is not yet common practice to have physicians or others address spiritual issues; patients may need an invitation to share their experiences. A spiritual history is simply a set of targeted questions aimed at inviting patients to share their spiritual or religious beliefs, and to guide them to delve into the meaning of life events.

The goal of each of these tools is to obtain a comprehensive understanding of a patient's relationship to spirituality, what the patient's spiritual beliefs are, and what his or her goals are for spiritual health. These tools are not meant for use as checklists, but rather to help give people the opportunity to share their beliefs, hopes, fears, and concerns. The spiritual history helps clinicians understand how the spirituality of patients influences their understanding of their illness and health, their coping with suffering, and their finding meaning in the midst of what is happening to them. The goals of the spiritual history are to:

- Invite patients to share spiritual and religious beliefs if they chose.
- Invite patients to define what spirituality is for them and their spiritual goals.
- Learn about the patient's beliefs and values.
- Assess for spiritual distress (meaninglessness, hopelessness) and spiritual resources of strength (hope, meaning and purpose, resiliency, spiritual community).

- Provide an opportunity for compassionate care whereby the health care professional connects to the patient in a deep and profound way.
- Empower the patient to find inner resources of healing and acceptance.
- Identify spiritual and religious beliefs that might affect health care decision making.
- Identify spiritual practices or rituals that might be helpful to incorporate into the treatment or care plan.

Preliminary questions can be used to address whether the patient wants to include a discussion of religion or spirituality in an explicit way. There are several tools that have been developed for this purpose. These include FICA (Puchalski & Romer, 2000; Puchalski, 2006a), SPIRIT (Maugans, 1996), and HOPE (Anandarajah & Hight, 2001) (see Appendix B). In addition, Nelson-Becker et al. (2006) developed a clinical assessment tool and domains of spiritual care for use by social workers (see figure 10). Generally these tools elicit more objective data (religious affiliation, spiritual identification, community, and spiritual practices) but also open the door to conversations about deeper and less measurable spiritual aspects such as meaning, importance of belief and/or faith, beliefs in afterlife, and sources of hope.

FIGURE 10   Clinical Assessment Tool

1. What helps you to experience a deep sense of meaning, purpose, and moral perspective in your life?

2. Is spirituality, religion, or faith important in your life? If so, please give examples. If not, please explain why they are not important, or, if you prefer, we do not need to discuss this further. (You can skip to Option 2 in question 4 below.)

3. If important to you, what terms for referring to spirituality, religion, or faith do you prefer?

4. Would you like to incorporate spirituality, religion, or faith in our work together? Please explain.

   —or—

   Option 2: (if the client is not comfortable with terms, "spirituality, religion, and faith") Would you like to incorporate the ways of experiencing meaning, purpose, or life satisfaction that you mentioned earlier? Please explain.

The areas of interest outlined in these tools are meant to serve as a guide for a discussion about spiritual issues. Questions can be customized to be consistent with the patient's or client's orientation and needs. For example, if the patient is coming for a routine visit, one might address spirituality in the context of stress management or health. If the patient has just been told of a serious diagnosis, then the questions might be phrased differently. For example, "Do you have spiritual beliefs that have helped you in difficult times before?" or "It must be hard to hear difficult news like this; do you have spiritual beliefs that might help you right now?"

As mentioned, the spiritual history is normally done during the social history section of the initial assessment as one is asking the patient about his or her living situation and significant relationships. The clinician can transition into how the person cares for himself or herself. Just as questions about exercise and how one deals with stress and difficult situations are an important part of self-care, questions about whether spiritual beliefs and practices are important to the patient should be included. The spiritual history might also be taken in specific clinical situations where spiritual issues may come up—for example, in breaking bad news or during end-of-life situations.

Recommendations

1. All patients should receive a simple and time-efficient spiritual screening at the point of entry into the health care system and appropriate referrals as needed.
2. Health care providers should adopt and implement structured assessment tools to facilitate documentation of needs and evaluation of outcomes of treatment.
3. All staff members should be vigilant, sensitive, and trained to recognize spiritual distress.
4. All health care professionals should be trained in doing a spiritual screening or history as part of their routine history and evaluation; unlicensed staff members should report all witnessed pain or spiritual distress.
5. Formal spiritual assessments should be made by a board-certified chaplain who should document their assessment and communicate

with the referring provider about their assessment and the plans of care.

6. Spiritual screenings, histories, and assessments should be communicated and documented in patient records (e.g., charts, computerized databases, and shared during interprofessional rounds). Documentation should be placed in a centralized location for use by all clinicians. If a computerized patient database is available, spiritual histories and assessments should be included.

7. Follow-up spiritual histories or assessments should be conducted for all patients whose medical, psychosocial, or spiritual condition changes and as part of routine follow-up in a medical history.

8. The chaplain should respond within twenty-four hours to a referral for spiritual assessment.

8 The Spiritual Treatment or Care Plan

Theoretical, Empirical, and Philosophical Background

Definition of Treatment/Care Plan

In the 1970s, George Engel (1977) laid out a vast alternative vision for health care when he described his biopsychosocial model. This model, not yet fully realized, placed the patient squarely within a nexus that included affective and other psychological states of a patient as a human person, as well as the significant interpersonal relationships that surround each person. At about the same time, White et al. (1996) was introducing an ecologic model of patient care that included attention to the patient's environment as well—a public health model of primary care. Neither of these models had anything to say about either spirituality or death. And while both models asserted certain truths about patients as human persons, neither provided any genuine grounding for these theories in what might be called a philosophical anthropology. That is to say, neither attempted to articulate a metaphysical grounding for their notions of patients as persons, although both seemed to depend on such a notion.

Both of these models have struggled to find a place in mainstream medicine. In large measure, this is because the successes of medicine have come about by embracing exactly the opposite model. Rather than considering the patient as a subject situated within a nexus of relationships, medical science has often considered the person as an object amenable to detached, disinterested investigation. Through the scientific reduction of the person to a specimen composed of systems, organs, cells, organelles, biochemical reactions, and the advance of genome medicine, there have been remarkable discoveries that have led to countless therapeutic advances. No one disputes that these advances have been good. But the experience of both patients and practitioners at the dawn of the twenty-first century is that the reductivist, scientific model is inadequate to the real needs of patients. Cracking the genetic code has not led us to understand who human beings are, what suffering and death mean, what may stand as a source of hope, what we mean by death with dignity, or what we may learn from seriously ill persons. All human persons have genomes, but human persons are not reducible to their genomes. To paraphrase Marcel (1949), a person is not a problem to be solved, but a mystery in which to dwell. To hold together in a single medical act both the reductionistic scientific truths that are so beneficial and also the larger truths about the patient as a human person is the really enormous challenge health care faces today.

The cornerstone of the philosophical anthropology we are proposing here is the concept of the human person as a being-in-relationship. Since each person is in relationship with transcendence, even if by way of rejecting the very possibility of transcendence, this means that human persons are intrinsically spiritual. From a philosophical point of view, one can argue that being *is* relationship. To know a thing (literally, any "thing") is to grasp the complex set of relationships that define it, whether that thing is a bacterium or a human being (Lonergan, 1958). This is all the more true of living things. Hans Jonas (2001) has put it this way:

> Being thus suspended in possibility is through and through a fact of polarity, and life always exhibits it in these basic respects: the polarity of being and not-being, of self and world, of form and matter, of freedom and necessity. These, as is easily seen, are forms of relation: life is essentially relationship; and relation as such implies "transcendence," a going-beyond-itself on the part of that which entertains the relation. (p. 4–5)

Disease can be described as a disruption of right relationships. It is not "looking at a bad body inside an otherwise healthy body." *Clostridium dificile* colitis is not a bad body that one sees under a microscope. The disease is not identical with the bacterium. Rather, the disease is a disturbance in the right relationships that constitute the unity and integrity of what we know to be a human being. A disease is always a disruption in right relationship.

Contemporary scientific healing retains the same formal structure that informed prescientific cultures—healing is still about the restora-

FIGURE 11   Illness and the Manifold of Relationships of the Patient as a Human Person

---

I. Intrapersonal:

  A. Physical relationships of body parts, organs, and physiological and biochemical processes

  B. Mind-body relationships—two-way interactions among symptoms, moods, and cognitive understandings and meanings and the person's physical state

---

I. Extrapersonal:

  A. Relationship with the physical environment

  B. Relationship with the interpersonal environment—family, friends, communities, political order

  C. Relationship with the transcendent

(Sulmasy, 2006)

tion of right relationships. However, this ought not to be limited to the restoration of the homeostatic relationships of the patient as an individual organism. Illness disturbs more than relationships *inside* the human organism. It disrupts families and workplaces. It shatters pre-existing patterns of coping. It raises questions about one's relationship with transcendence.

Thus, one can say that illness disturbs relationships both inside and outside the body of the human person. Inside the body, the disturbances are twofold—(a) the relationships between and among the various body parts and biochemical processes and (b) the relationship between the mind and the body. Outside the body, these disturbances are also twofold—(a) the relationship between the individual patient and his or her environment, including the ecological, physical, familial, social, and political nexus of relationships surrounding the patient, and (b) the relationship between the patient and the transcendent. (See figure 11.)

In biopsychosocial-spiritual model, healing can be defined even more precisely than by the vague references one sometimes hears to "making whole." Healing, in its most basic sense, means the restoration of right relationships. What genuinely holistic health care means is a system of health care that attends to all of the disturbed relationships of the ill person as a whole, restoring those that can be restored, even if the person is not thereby completely restored to perfect wholeness. A holistic approach to healing means the correction of the physiologic disturbances and the restoration of the *milieu interior* is only the beginning of the task. Holistic healing requires attention to the psychological, social, and spiritual disturbances as well. As Teilhard de Chardin (1960) put it: besides the *milieu interior*, there is also a *milieu divine*. Furthermore, this means that even when cure is no longer possible, when the *milieu interior* can no longer be restored, healing is still possible, and the healing professions still have a role. Healing is the crux of what spirituality attends to … the *milieu divine*—the healing of the whole person and not just the body. As Remen noted: "We thought we could cure everything, but it turns out we can only cure a small amount of human suffering. The rest of it needs to be healed" (Tippet, 2007, p. 213).

No matter what the patient's spiritual history, serious illness raises for the patient questions about the value and meaning of the patient's life, suffering, and death. These are the obvious questions— those about meaning, value, and relationship (Sulmasy, 1999, 2000, 2001). The attention to these questions affords for patients the opportunity to reflect on the broader aspect of their life and on the spiritual dimension within that can open up to the possibility of healing.

So the appropriate care of seriously ill persons requires attention to the restoration of all the intrapersonal and extrapersonal relationships that can still be addressed, even when the patient is dying. Considering the relationship between mind and body in its broadest sense, symptomatic treatment restores the human person by relieving him or her of the experiences of pain, nausea, dyspnea, fatigue, anxiety, and depression. Considering the relationship between the human person and the environment, this means, for example, that the facilitation of reconciliation with family and friends is genuine healing within the biopsychosocial-spiritual model. For the seriously ill individual experiencing love, being understood as valuable even when no longer economically productive, and accepting the role of teacher by providing valuable lessons to those who provide the care, are all experiences of healing. Finally, when questions about existence, meaning, value, and relationship arise in the context of health care, they are starkly circumscribed by the finitude that disease, injury, and death make manifest. Healing, in a complete sense, must involve the overriding question of whether the answers to these perennial questions transcend that finitude.

Michael was dying from lung and colon cancer. While struggling with these cancers for many years, his one hope was to have a relationship with God. He felt that he understood intellectually what that was, but he wanted the emotional and spiritual experience of God. One office visit I (Puchalski) had taught him the relaxation response. As he was focusing on a word that was spiritual for him, he began to cry about three minutes into the breathing exercise. When we finished he told me that the tears were tears of joy. In all his years of meditating, he had never felt what happened to him that day. In his words he felt "healed even though I am dying." Healing can be manifested in so many different ways ... body, mind, and spirit.

If the human person is essentially a being-in-relationship, even the person who has chosen to believe that there is no such thing as transcendence has made his or her choice in relationship to that question. Each person must live and die according to the answer each gives to the question of whether life or death has a meaning that transcends both life and death. In the biopsychosocial-spiritual model, the facilitation of a patient's grappling with such questions is a way to approach healing.

Applying the Biopsychosocial-Spiritual Model of Care

Everyone, according to the biopsychosocial-spiritual model, has a spiritual history. For many people, this spiritual history unfolds within the context of an explicit religious tradition; for others it unfolds within the context of nature, relationships, or values. But regardless of how it has unfolded, this spiritual history helps shape each patient as a whole person, and when life-threatening illness strikes, it strikes

FIGURE 12   The Biopsychosocial-Spiritual Model of Care at the End of Life

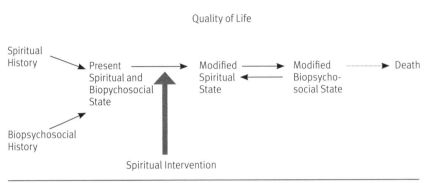

(Daaelman & Hanson, 2008)

each person in his or her totality (Ramsey, 1970). This totality includes not simply the biologic, psychological, and social aspects of the person (Engel, 1992), but the spiritual aspects of the whole person as well (King, 2000; Mckee & Chappel, 1992). The biopsychosocial-spiritual model is not a "dualism" in which a "soul" accidentally inhabits a body. Rather, in this model, the biologic, psychological, social, and spiritual are only distinct dimensions of the person, and no one aspect can be disaggregated from the whole. Each aspect can be affected differently by a person's history and illness, and can interact and affect other aspects of the person.

Figure 12 schematically represents how a few selected aspects of spirituality that health care researchers have been able to measure can be viewed in relation to the patient who is approached by a chaplain, nurse, physician, or other member of the team, with an eye toward some sort of spiritual intervention. This diagram is obviously an oversimplification and does not fully account for the dynamic and iterative processes that constitute a spiritual life. However, as a rough approximation, it can help to illustrate some important features clinicians and researchers ought to bear in mind. Patients come to the clinical encounter with spiritual and biopsychosocial histories. Their lives have been deeply influenced by what has transpired before. They come to the moment of encounter with the health care professional already having personalities, virtues and vices, religious or other spiritual practices, and styles of coping that may be religious or not. The quality of a patient's life at the moment of encounter is not only affected by his or her physical and psychological state, but also by his or her spiritual state. At that moment the clinician approaches, hoping to assist the patient spiritually. That encounter (whether directly intended as an "intervention" or not) will affect the patient's spiritual state. That spiritual state is in dynamic relationship with the entirety of the patients' integrated self—biologically, psychologically, and socially. This new state constitutes part of the quality of living that the patient's experiences in the time leading up to death (and in the view of many spiritual traditions whatever lies beyond death as well). This simple picture must not be taken too literally. The encounter depicted in the figure must be understood as something that happens in the course of many "interventions" by many individuals (or on multiple occasions through repeated encounters with the same individual). Spirituality is dynamic, not static.

Formulation of Spiritual Goals

As spiritual issues are assessed in the clinical setting, patients and families should be empowered to formulate spiritual goals. Goals for spiritual care are patient-centered in that they are dictated by the patient or family member. They can be mutually agreed on in the sense of a "contract" or may develop over time as life events transpire. It can be both therapeutic and important to identify these goals. For patients, it can be therapeutic for the individual to identify and prioritize those questions that are personally most important or distressing. This can help provide reassurance to patients that their spiritual concerns have been heard and a plan is in place to address them. It may also send a message that someone in the health care area not only is accountable for addressing the patient's spiritual concerns, but will accompany him in the process of meeting these goals.

Determination of spiritual goals should include not only the potential for growth of an individual (or their weaknesses) but their strengths and degree of internal resiliency. It is useful to use a theoretical framework to structure the process of setting goals. The framework should be comprehensive and focus on a "whole person" approach. Many models for comprehensive evaluation examine domains such as values, vocation, social support, creativity, transcendence, physical functioning, ethnic and cultural considerations, and psychological considerations (Anandarajah & Hight, 2001; Fitchett, 2002; Galek et al., 2005; Hodge, 2001; Puchalski & Romer, 2000; Skalla & McCoy, 2006). Goals focused on bolstering strengths and addressing interpersonal growth may facilitate a deepened sense of spirituality; an enhanced appreciation for life both in the sense of its fragility and uncertainty, as well as its inherent value; a reordering of life priorities; increased empathy and compassion for others; increased self-esteem; and a greater sense of meaning in life. When successfully negotiated, the journey can expand a person's repertoire of thoughts and actions to be able to engage in new ways of thinking and behaving creatively and help people to see coherence in life events to foster a belief in how full of meaning life is (Jim et al., 2006). Goals focused on potential areas of growth may focus on a sense of meaninglessness, for example. Meaninglessness may contribute to decreased motivation or depression. Statements such as "Life is hopeless" or "I can't do anything about this" may reflect lack of meaning for the individual to structure his or her life into a new normal. A goal might be to assist the patient in finding meaning using a variety of interventions such as journaling or life review.

From the perspective of the spiritual care provider, goals should be as specific as possible to be measurable with respect to outcomes. Measuring goals can be done with something as simple as a visual analogue scale (VAS). For example, a patient struggling with hopelessness might cocreate the treatment plan by making specific goals about finding hope. This goal might be measured using a VAS scored from one to ten that asks the patient to what degree he or she find hope. This measure can be repeated over time to assess progress and determine what level of progress is acceptable and realistic to the patient. A different patient might discover during the spiritual history that he or she wants to develop a spiritual practice. The plan would be to refer him or her to appropriate resources for finding a practice that meets his or her spiritual needs. Progress can be measured by specific outcomes, such as whether the person is able to find and maintain a practice on a daily basis. The measure will depend on the type of spiritual goal chosen. Progress toward goals can indicate effectiveness of an intervention.

Referrals

While we have argued that all clinicians have an obligation to elicit patients' spiritual needs and respect patients' beliefs and struggles, this does not imply that the clinician must be the one who provides specific spiritual care. All clinicians have a moral obligation to recognize the limits of their expertise. When the care requirements are beyond the scope of competence of the attending practitioner, that practitioner must refer to colleagues who are competent to provide what is needed. The virtue associated with this duty is humility. This is thought to be the point of the dictum of the Hippocratic Oath, "I will not use the knife, not even on sufferers from stone, but will withdraw in favor of such men as are engaged in this work." The Hippocratic practitioners were not experts in this most dangerous of ancient surgical interventions, but knew there were specialists who had that competency. Likewise, clinicians should generally limit their attention to patients' spirituality to an assessment of their spiritual concerns and needs and a respect for them as whole people struggling with spiritual questions. They should not engage in significant spiritual counseling for patients, since this is beyond their expertise. Further, even if a particular clinician were to acquire the necessary expertise (e.g., pursuing a degree in pastoral counseling), there are still good ethical reasons why physicians and nurses should not engage in spiritual therapy but should refer to chaplains or the patient's own personal clergy. There are, for example, some things a patient might want to tell the physician that he or she might not want to tell the clergy, and vice versa. Without a clear separation of roles, a patient who was providing a spiritual history to a nurse might be uncertain whether the medical information was useful or merely a confession. Therefore, while we would hold that clinicians have an obligation to engage the spiritual aspects of illness, death, and dying, we are not advocating a form of neoshamanism in which the roles of religious figure and healer are completely intertwined. A team care approach to the spiritual care of the sick and the dying is needed. Excellent spiritual care can be thought of as a circular process in which initial screening by clinicians leads to referrals to spiritual care providers who in turn conduct in-depth assessments and develop a plan of spiritual care, which is then shared with the team.

As an example, an elderly man was admitted to hospice and recognized to be extremely angry and hostile and reluctant to accept help for the team. While he acknowledged being an atheist and adamantly refused to be seen by the chaplain, the nurse continued to allow the patient to "rage" until the point when the patient had developed such a trusting relationship with the nurse that he admitted that as he now faced death, he was not only beginning to believe in a higher power, but also he was very regretful for his lifelong avoidance of religion and criticism of believers. Chaplaincy intervention was critical at this time of spiritual distress, but it was also essential that all team members were aware of this distress and were open to his need to verbalize his regret over previous beliefs and evolution to a new acceptance of a transcendent force.

Spiritual Interventions

Spiritual interventions include a variety of activities and processes such as spiritual counseling, encouraging patients to utilize already established spiritual practices (e.g., prayer, meditation), participation in spiritual or faith communities, meaning-centered therapy, dignity therapy, journaling, and participation in the arts. In prescribing or suggesting a spiritual intervention, ultimately it is our goal as clinicians to promote spiritual well-being. Increased attention has been paid to designing spiritual care interventions such as listening to patient's personal stories (O'Conner & Wicker, 1995), meaning-making interventions, and short-term life review (Ando et al., 2008; Breitbart, 2003; Lee et al., 2006).

There has been some controversy over whether religious or spiritual interventions should be prescribed. Waldfogel and Wolpe (1993) noted that "although religious interventions are not substitutes for therapeutic interventions, 'religious prescriptions' are ethically sound and may complement more traditional therapies." We would caution against prescribing religious interventions unless the clinician knows that that particular intervention is something the patient has used in the past and it is acceptable to that patient.

There are some spiritual therapeutic models that have been developed and studied. One is the Dignity-Conserving Practices Model by Chochinov (2002 and 2006) and Chochinov et al. (2004). Dignity-conserving practices refer to various personal approaches or techniques patients use to bolster or maintain their sense of dignity. Three components of these practices are:

1. Living in the moment (focusing on immediate issues in the service of not worrying about the future).
2. Maintaining normalcy (continuous or routine behaviors, which help individuals manage day-to-day challenges).
3. Seeking spiritual comfort (turning toward or finding solace in one's religious or spiritual belief system).

The other spiritual therapeutic model in psycho-oncology is meaning-centered psychotherapy for patients with cancer (Chochinov and Breitbart, 2009). In this model, the investigators had patients participate in eight sessions of group therapy focused on how they find meaning in the midst of their illness. Both of these models have been studied. There are also models of group spiritual direction facilitated by spiritual directors that may be applicable to the clinical setting.

Kissane et al. (2001) asserted that demoralization syndrome, with its attendant hopelessness and loss of meaning, represents an important expression of existential distress in palliative care patients. They advocate a broad range of approaches for hopelessness, loss of meaning, and existential distress experiences by palliative patients. These include (a) providing continuity of care and active symptom management, (b) exploring patients' attitudes toward hope and meaning in life, (c) balancing support for grief with promotion of hope, (d) fostering the search for a renewed purpose and role in life, (e) using cognitive therapy to reframe negative beliefs, (f) involving pastoral or spiritual care for spiritual support, (g) promoting supportive relationships and use of volunteers, (h) enhancing family functioning by conducting family meetings, and (i) reviewing the goals of care in multidisciplinary team settings.

Mind-Body Interventions   The mind has tremendous potential to affect how a person perceives life, stress, illness, dying, and the world. There are a number of studies on meditation and other spiritual and religious practices that demonstrate a positive physical response, especially in relation to levels of stress hormones and modulation of the stress response (Benson, 1996; Seeman et al., 2003). The data demonstrate an association between meditation and some spiritual or religious practices and certain physiologic processes, including cardiovascular, neuroendocrine, and immune function. These studies show a significant role for mind-body interventions in stress management and as an adjunct to treatment of chronic illness and end-of-life symptoms. For example, pain and dyspnea may effectively be managed by meditation or the relaxation response. The clear connection between stress and deregulation of immune function and the hypothalamic-pituitary-adrenal axis has been established, creating a theoretical basis for how stress can lead to diseases (Ader et al., 1995; McEwen, 1998; McEwen & Stellar, 1993).

Spiritual beliefs and mindfulness help people tap into their own inherent abilities to heal and cope, find meaning and purpose and hope, and do well with whatever life offers them. By focusing on the physical aspects of care, health care professionals and, as a result, the systems in which they operate often neglect the very areas that research is now beginning to find critical to care. Such approaches allow for the recognition of people's ability to transcend suffering and offer opportunities for health care professionals to treat the whole person—body and mind. It has been generally accepted that spiritual practices such as prayer, meditation, yoga, tai chi, among many others, counteract chronic stress effects on the body and rebalance autonomic nervous system and HPA axis. Reports of their use are appearing in mainstream journals and moving into the clinical research arena. The growing body of evidence supports the use of these practices as adjunctive modalities to medical management of chronic conditions such as pain and elevated blood pressure (Schneider et al., 2005; Puchalski, 2006b).

Spiritual Counseling   The spiritual dimension of care is the fundamental act of "being with" another in need, healing through facilitating wholeness. Spiritual care does not require completion in one session but may evolve over time and can encompass both pastoral or spiritual care and more directed spiritual counseling. Spiritual counseling is done by the board-certified chaplain, clergy, or pastoral counselor. Spiritual counseling is a step forward out of the immediate moment of the situation and ideally builds on the pastoral or spiritual care that has already been received. It is dictated by the needs and goals of the patient or caregiver. As patients and their caregivers face life-threatening or serious illness, they must negotiate some of the most spiritually threatening questions central to human existence. They can respond either positively (spiritual growth) or negatively (spiritual distress) to this threat. Spiritual care begins by addressing distress and is a fundamental act of "being with." In a moment of crisis or distress, a person may have the need to be accompanied in that pain. As the immediate crisis passes, questions repeatedly important to patients are: Why is this happening to me? What is the meaning of my life? What happens when we die? (Miller, 2005). When patients are ready to move forward, spiritual counseling may facilitate the transition toward healing and spiritual growth as the patient actively and intentionally seeks to answer these types of questions. Identifying which type of spiritual care, pastoral care, and pastoral counseling is necessary must occur and depends on the patient or caregiver goals.

In noncrisis situations spiritual issues may come up that also require counseling. Just as in psychological counseling, very often the spiritual history or assessment itself will lead the patient to an understanding of his or her spiritual concerns, which is comforting to his or her and which can be affirmed by the counselor. Many patients know what they believe but may be concerned if they conceive these beliefs to be divergent from the norm for their faith tradition and therefore "wrong." Affirmation from the counselor that beliefs are acceptable may be all the person needs to enlist these beliefs in their coping process. For example, a young adult diagnosed with a brain tumor shared tremendous angst in reporting on the spiritual assessment that he had left the Catholic Church, which had been his family's religious affiliation for three generations, and had become involved with what he described as a "liberal, more modern" church. Through ongoing counseling with both a social worker and chaplain, the man was able to recognize that while his leaving the Catholic Church had caused great conflict with his parents, he still believed strongly that it was the right decision and that his new religious community offered tremendous support and meaning.

There are several core concepts integral to spiritual counseling. First, a diagnosis of life-threatening illness may affect the core personhood of an individual in a variety of ways. The body of literature describing how people respond continues to grow. Some may integrate the diagnosis as part of life and resume normal behavior patterns and activities (Vachon, 2008). Many identify the diagnosis as a crisis. Regardless, this period of time in a person's life can provide an opportunity for spiritual transformation (Cole et al., 2007) and growth (Jaarsma et al., 2006; Steel et al., 2008; Tedeschi & Calhoun, 1996). During this period, a person's entire identity may come into question and be redesigned during the process of redefining his or her personal sense of self. Some may find themselves forced to reorder goals and priorities because of physical disability or role changes. Alternatively they may choose this reordering and find themselves motivated in new ways or toward new opportunities (Vachon, 2008). Still others may struggle to derive a sense of meaning or purpose in their illness experience in order to redefine or reframe their faith in a higher power. The positive response to life-threatening illness has been greater confidence and assertiveness (McGrath, 2004), translating to less dependence on others and a greater ability to assert personal needs with an increased awareness of physical needs. Interpersonal outcomes included helping patients to be less judgmental and more compassionate, having a desire to live life to the fullest, reevaluating work values, and developing a stronger connection with family and friends. Lastly, they had a sense of increased respect from others. These positive outcomes demonstrate considerable spiritual growth that can inform the process of setting spiritual goals to build solid core resiliency in the context of counseling.

The second core concept in spiritual counseling is the process of making meaning from the illness experience. This process can have a profound impact on spiritual growth. Finding meaning in events, especially suffering, seems to be a central element in good coping (Park & Folkman, 1997). Religious or spiritual meanings are common choices (Spilka et al., 1985). Meaning includes "one's sense of purpose in life, the belief in the value of life, the coherent explanation of life events, well-being, and spirituality" (Jim et al., 2006, p. 1360). Therefore, meaning in this context can be defined as having many components and is present when one has a sense of purpose, coherence, and fulfillment in a life that is perceived to have value (Jim et al., 2006).

These components, spiritual beliefs, spiritual practices, and the construction of meanings grounded in a relationship with a source that is perceived as sacred (McGrath, 2004) can act synergistically to create meaning. It is the content and context of meaning that are important to quality of life, not simply the idea of having meaning (Clarke, 2006).

Functionally, coping and spirituality are both meaning-centered processes that involve a search for significance in life events. Park and Folkman (1997) identify two specific types of meaning. "Global" meaning represents beliefs about the order of life or the universe as well as personal life goals and purpose. "Situational" meaning, in contrast, is the interaction of a person's global beliefs within the context of a particular life experience. When a person undergoes a stressful life experience, his or her ability to find congruence between the two types of meaning determines whether or not that person feels stressed (Jim et al., 2006). Therefore, meaning-making is the response to the impulse for congruence. The ability to find situational meaning in the illness experience that is congruent with patients' global meaning has been associated with better adjustment and subsequently less spiritual distress.

Many spiritual practices are used in the process of making-meaning. Patients have reported regular use of spirituality and religion to cope with their diagnosis and treatment (Jim et al., 2006) and find spiritual comfort by perceiving the experience of illness in terms of a positive spiritual journey (McGrath, 2004; Rancour, 2008). The journey metaphor includes concepts such as everything happens for a reason, having a sense of being "chosen" for this experience, the need to see illness as a challenge and take personal responsibility to overcome that challenge, and having a sense of personal growth and pride in meeting that challenge (McGrath, 2004). This metaphor can be used in spiritual counseling to reframe life experiences and facilitate congruence of meaning for a person facing serious illness of end of life and who is experiencing spiritual distress.

In modern spiritual counseling, the goal is to help the sufferer find a meaning that promotes positive coping rather than imposing a meaning that conforms to the generally accepted belief system of the person's faith tradition. Attention needs to be paid not only to the content of the belief, but also its affective component and function for the individual. Individuals who believe God has caused their illness may be in great distress because the illness means to them that God is punishing them, or they may be comforted because they take the illness as a sign that God is in control. Many Muslims believe that while suffering is sent by Allah, it is an opportunity to atone for some of their sins and, therefore, they have a better chance of entering heaven. Persons providing the spiritual counseling need to take extreme care not to impose their own meaning on the patient's beliefs, but attend closely to how a particular belief functions for this particular person.

The third concept important to spiritual counseling is transition. Transition theory (Bridges, 2004) has been used to provide structure when talking to patients about how to remake their life into a new normal (Rancour, 2008); this theory describes three stages of transition. The first stage, "endings," is characterized by letting go of old relationships (with health care providers) and roles (an ill person), even if the transition is positive. This implies a process of grief, sadness, and anger as this stage is left behind. Support for this mourning comes from "being with," which is a central component of pastoral care rather than "fixing." The effort to experience and tolerate the patient's most difficult emotions will allow the individual to heal and move on rather than remain stuck in their own distress. Jim was devastated when the doctor told him he had lung cancer. His first reaction was denial and his second was guilt about smoking. The week following the news was filled with panic, anxiety, and emptiness. Jim realized life would never be the same and that one day he would die from this illness. His doctor spent time listening to Jim's feelings and was present to his suffering. His doctor did not try to remove the suffering or "fix him"; she just accepted Jim where he was and supported him in his journey. She listened to his beliefs. She asked him about sources of hope in the midst of his despair. She encouraged him to journal about his feelings. Eventually Jim found acceptance. He accepted the suffering as normal and the uncertainty as part of life's journey. Jim was able to find a way to live with his cancer, to live with hope as well as despair, and to find new meaning in his life. Over time he found that his own suffering enabled him to be truly compassionate to others in ways he was never before in his life. His cancer to him became a gift to a deeper and more meaningful life.

The second stage, or "neutral zone," is characterized by a sense of confusion, chaos, and anxiety. This stage is characterized by a lack of structure. Patients are struggling to define a new normal. In that process, a loss of identity can trigger discomfort, anxiety, and panic. They need to be assured that their feelings are normal and that the new identity will emerge once it is formed. Encouraging patients to attend to this distress by "caring for themselves" will allow them to tolerate suffering within themselves that can later translate into compassion for others. Cultivating silence and reflection on the emerging identity through journaling, meditating, or use of ritual may be helpful. Finally, a "new beginning" stage is reached where survivors are ready to move on and take advantage of new opportunities. It is important to resist trying to "fix" in this stage also and instead assist the patient to identify new skills, ask about new life meaning, and try new things (Rancour, 2008).

Transformational processes toward spiritual growth can be both powerful and painful; therefore, it is the responsibility of those who care for patients at the end of life to support the experience of that process and find ways to facilitate spiritual growth. The provision of spiritual counseling can be a critical piece of that responsibility, so it is important that spiritual counseling be undertaken by someone with specific training in pastoral care, ideally a board-certified chaplain or pastoral counselor. This is entirely appropriate because of the specialized knowledge and role of the clinically trained and board-certified chaplain. Other providers of spiritual counseling, however, may include psychiatrists or psychologists, social workers, physicians, or advanced practice nurses who have received education in pastoral or spiritual counseling and who have appropriate supervisory relationships that support their practice of spiritual counseling.

Spiritual Practice and Rituals   Spiritual distress and existential suffering are multifaceted and can be caused, in part, by disease and illness, social isolation, and feeling cut off from the normal events of everyday living. One way patients and families may find meaning and comfort as they navigate the journey of life-threatening illness is through spiritual practice and rituals (Bryson, 2004).

Spiritual practices are those activities one undertakes to express that deep inner meaning that represents the core of our being and are capable of uniting us with the transcendent (Puchalski & O'Donnell, 2005; Puchalski et al., 2004). Spiritual practices promote well-being, coping, growth, and relationships (Taylor, 2001). Spiritual practices can range from religious practices and attendance at religious services to more broadly defined spiritual practices such as prayer, meditation, sacred or inspirational reading, journaling, reflection, intentional appreciation of beauty, or finding peace in nature.

Prayer, meditation, and visualization most clearly illustrate the overlap among the traditional practice of pastoral care, modern spiritual care, and treatment techniques normally classed as "psychological." As the concept of what constitutes prayer has moved from prescripted formulations often only said during a service of worship to any communication between a person and what he or she conceives to be a higher power, the definitions of prayer and meditation have clearly converged. While prayer is generally conceived as a dialogue where the person both speaks and listens, meditation and visualization put the practitioner more clearly in a listening or receiving mode. Benson and Proctor (1984) pointed out that religious language functions as an effective focus for meditation if the words have meaning for the person involved. They also found that there are beneficial outcomes to repetitive actions such as using a mantra in meditation, saying the rosary, or focusing on a phrase or word in meditation.

Today many spiritual caregivers use meditation and visualization focused on religious, spiritual images and words, or images from the arts, nature, or music as one of their treatment options. Christianity, Judaism, and Islam share the Psalms, which can readily be used for various types of meditation and support expression of a full range of emotion. One might also use poetry or other inspirational texts. The experienced spiritual caregiver can assist the religious or spiritual patient to find appropriate words or images to use in a meditation or visualization as well as expanding the patient's concept of prayer to make it more useful in coping.

Ritual has been defined as "the established form for a ceremony" or "a ceremonial act or action" (Ritual, 2008). Moore (1996) wrote that rituals are "any actions that speak to the soul and to the deep imagination, whether or not it all has practical effects.... Even the smallest rites of everyday existence are important to the soul." Rituals embody symbolic meaning, punctuate experience into meaningful chunks of time (e.g., life transitions), help people address that which existentially remains ambiguous or "mystery," and help facilitate a mystical expression such as an encounter with God, the divine or transcendent energy within a ritual (Griffith & Griffith, 2002).

Just as the definition of prayer has broadened to encompass a wider range of behaviors, ritual has been redefined to make it more useful for a wider range of patients. Probably because its mechanism of action is not clearly understood, the power of ritual has been vastly underestimated, especially in coping with suffering and loss. However, people seem to turn to ritual as a way to cope. An example of a ritual that has been used in palliative care is a reconciliation ritual. When reviewing their life history, many patients have issues of guilt, shame, or the need to reconcile with self, others, or God. Such a ritual can be very beneficial for patients. Other rituals include honoring the patient, religious rituals and rites, and blessings. Spiritual care providers may ask patients about rituals that have been a part of their spiritual lives as well as suggest rituals that may have meaning at this time.

Ritual in spiritual care can fall into at least two categories. The first encompasses set rituals from the person's faith tradition. Sufferers often return to rituals of their childhood religion even when they have otherwise disavowed it. The mother of a teenaged boy newly diagnosed with cancer who had converted from Roman Catholicism to Protestantism many years before because the rituals had no meaning for her asked the chaplain to have a Catholic priest bless her son with holy water. A Jewish patient who practiced his faith as a child but who had not done so for most of his life began to cry when a traditional prayer for healing was said in Hebrew. A Muslim patient was upset because he was unable to perform the physical movements that accompany his daily prayer. Many patients attend worship in their faith tradition regularly and feel extremely uneasy when they are unable to do so.

The second category of rituals are personal rituals that people have designed for themselves as expressions of their spiritual beliefs, longings, or values. An example would be a ritual of offering up the names of one's patient to a higher being or energy force as a way of a health care professional's recognition that he or she is limited in what he or she can do for the patient. Or a family may have a ritual around a meal or special event that is unique to that family and not necessarily of a religious or cultural tradition. Or a patient may have developed a ritual using symbols from nature that bring peace to that person or connects him or her to this or her inner life.

Caregivers need to carefully assess what rituals might be important to patients in maintaining the feeling of normalcy in their lives or in giving them a sense of control over their situation. Many patients have set daily schedules for prayer, reading, and religious ritual that are important to maintain. When the patient is unable to perform a normal ritual because of his or her physical state or a hospital regulation, a chaplain may be helpful in creating a comparable ritual. In the case of the Muslim patient, the Imam was able to modify the ritual so that imaging the movements in the patient's mind while praying was equivalent in the eyes of Allah to actually doing them. A Roman Catholic patient who cannot swallow may be comforted by the assurance that his or her intention to receive the Eucharist will be seen by God as equivalent to the actual act. It is important to determine which rituals that are important to the family members must be done by a clergyperson of his or her faith tradition and which can be done by the family or a spiritual care provider. Reconciliation rituals, for example, normally only have power for the patient if they are done by a clergyperson of his or her faith tradition. As patients in health care institutions become sicker and less able to attend worship services of their faith, substitutes like services on individual nursing units or over in-house television become increasing critical.

End-of-life rituals are also extremely important to many patients and their loved ones. Staff should carefully assess with the family members what rituals they will want to have performed so proper preparations can be made. Many such rituals involve candles or incense, which are not safe to use in the hospital setting or even at home if oxygen is in use. A chaplain can help the family find an accommodation that will allow the ritual to be performed safely.

It is often important to be able to improvise rituals to deal with specific circumstances. In the recovery of bodies from the World Trade Center, complex rituals evolved for the handling of each body that, on one hand, slowed the excavation process, but, on the other hand, assured all involved that each body was handled with respect. Many neonatal units have developed ritualized procedures that help parents begin to grieve. Van der Hart (1988) has written extensively about devising particular rituals especially for coping with specific losses.

A study by Tatsumura et al. (2003) found patients with cancer use various internal and external resources that they called spiritual practices including personal faith, individual prayer, relationship or dialogue with God, religious texts, attending religious services, and meditation. Other practices include finding and spending time at locations of spiritual energy, including churches, specific geographic locations, or certain natural settings (Van der Hart, 2008). Rituals can be religious in nature and thousands of years old, or they can be created by an individual in the present moment to acknowledge or honor a situation or event. Rituals and practices, such as saying the rosary or chanting, might be identified as religious in nature, while a person who walks the labyrinth or does mindfulness meditation might refer to his or her practice as spiritual. Professionals should respect any spiritual practices important to the patient, be it prayer, meditation, reflection, listening to certain music, enjoying solitude, writing poetry, or journaling. One can then incorporate these practices as appropriate. Patients and families with life-threatening illnesses who are being cared for in acute hospitals or long-term care facilities may feel disconnected from the world as they know it and all that is familiar (Bryson, 2004). The NCP Guidelines (2009) call for the patient and family to be encouraged to use and display any religious or spiritual symbols meaningful to them and for the palliative care team to support or facilitate spiritual rituals or practices desired by the patient/family unit, especially at the time of death. Professionals can facilitate the possibility of easing patients' distress and suffering by encouraging them to utilize and display their own religious or spiritual symbols, supporting them in their own spiritual practices, and facilitating and advocating for meaningful rituals to help to reconnect them to themselves, their family, and the transcendent.

In recommending any of these practices, clinicians must adhere to the ethical guidelines. Prayer or a religious text should not be recommended to patients who are not religious. Guided imagery and rituals should be congruent with the patients' beliefs systems, not those of the health care professionals. When recommending a ritual, the clinician should refer to the information a patient shares during a spiritual history. If a patient identifies a ritual as important, the clinician can ask whether that ritual might be helpful in the particular clinical situation the patient is in. A clinician could ask, "In the past, meditation has helped you. Do you think it might be helpful now?" It is generally recommended to rely on trained spiritual care professionals in selecting which spiritual treatment option is best for patients.

Practice Principles

Spiritual issues, once identified, need to be integrated into the patients' overall treatment or care plan. After identifying spiritual issues or spiritual distress through a spiritual history or assessment, clinicians can determine what the treatment plans should be. In the ideal setting, as part of the team, nonchaplain clinicians could discuss their findings from the history with the chaplains and cocreate a treatment plan. In cases where the chaplain is not readily available, the clinicians should still identify the issues and then consider appropriate referrals to chaplain, pastoral counselors, spiritual directors, or therapists.

As with any medical assessment and plan, the first step after communicating with patients about spiritual issues is to diagnose the problems. Spiritual issues can be organized in terms of diagnoses. In this case, physicians, advanced practice nurses, and physician assistants can make these diagnoses. Chaplains would reaffirm these basic diagnoses, change the diagnosis of the nonchaplain clinician, and/or make other diagnoses based on more advanced spiritual assessment. The model for diagnoses of spiritual issues can be similar to that used for psychiatric diagnosis by a primary care clinician, in what might be called a generalist-specialist model. A patient can be diagnosed with depression by the primary care clinician, and the psychiatrist then diagnoses the type of depression and any other associated diagnoses that may be affecting that diagnosis. For example, the psychiatrist might then diagnose depression with psychotic features with borderline personality disorder, complicating the diagnosis in the patient referred to this psychiatrist by the primary care physician. A physician might diagnose a patient with conflicted belief systems and refer to a chaplain. The chaplain, during his or her detailed assessment, may uncover concerns with the patient's relationship with deity and meaninglessness as a result of that concern.

The clinician would use a spiritual history tool to:

1. Identify spiritual issues
   a. Distress or needs
   b. Hopes
   c. Resources (sense of the sacred or significant, community, positive religious or spiritual coping, meaning)
   d. Beliefs affecting health care decision making
2. Develop spiritual goal (if applicable)
3. Formulate a treatment plan based on the issues and goals, determining and implementing appropriate spiritual interventions (spiritual counseling, spiritual practices, rituals, reading materials [spiritual or philosophical], meaning-centered therapy, dignity therapy, spiritual legacy building, storytelling, journaling, music, arts, and mind-body interventions such relaxation response)
4. Refer to appropriate spiritual care professionals

Diagnosis of Spiritual Issue

Health care professionals determine how to integrate information from the spiritual assessment into the patient's overall treatment plan. Using the language consistent with practice in most health care settings, this includes identifying or diagnosing the spiritual problems/needs; identifying spiritual goals (if appropriate); and determining, implementing, and evaluating the appropriate spiritual interventions (see figure 13, table 7, 8, and 9 in section below). Health care professionals involved in assessing and referring patients should identify spiritual issues or make spiritual diagnoses if applicable. Some spiritual diagnosis labels currently exist, but these may be limited in scope (e.g., to patients with cancer) and also are not presently used for reimbursement. The nursing diagnostic nomenclature defines spiritual distress as "impaired ability to experience and integrate meaning and purpose in life through connectedness with self, other, art, music, literature, nature, and/or power greater than oneself." Related nursing diagnoses may include inability to practice religious ritual, conflict between religious and spiritual beliefs and prescribed health regimen, loss of faith, anger at God, guilt over "sins," and discontinuation of religious practices (NANDA-I, 2009).

The National Comprehensive Cancer Network (2008) Practice Guidelines in Oncology describe the following spiritual diagnostic codes:

- Grief
- Concerns about afterlife
- Conflicted or challenged belief systems
- Loss of faith
- Concerns with meaning and purpose of life
- Concerns with relationship with deity
- Isolation from religious community
- Guilt
- Hopelessness
- Conflict between religious beliefs and recommended treatments
- Ritual needs

There is a diagnosis coding for mental health professionals to use when a spiritual issue is diagnosed. This category can be used when the focus of clinical attention is a religious or spiritual problem (e.g., distressing experiences that involve loss or questioning of faith, problems associated with conversion to a new faith, or questioning of other spiritual values that may not necessarily be related to an organized church or religious institution). These religious or spiritual problems can be coded on Axis I as problem only Problem *and* unrelated mental disorder Problem *and* related mental disorder, or Problem leading to mental disorder leading to the spiritual problem (American Psychiatric Association, 2000).

In summary, a clinician may identify spiritual distress that is a spiritual diagnosis or a clinician may identify a spiritual issue or resource of strength that does not meet the criteria for a spiritual diagnosis. In general a spiritual issue becomes a diagnosis if the following criteria are met:

1. The spiritual issue leads to distress or suffering (e.g., lack of meaning, conflicted religious beliefs, inability to forgive).
2. The spiritual issue is the cause of a psychological or physical diagnosis such as depression, anxiety, or acute or chronic pain (e.g., severe meaninglessness that leads to depression or suicidality, guilt that leads to chronic physical pain).

3. The spiritual issue is a secondary cause or affects the presenting psychological or physical diagnosis (e.g., hypertension is difficult to control because the patient refuses to take medications because of his or her religious beliefs).

Kathy is a thirty-year-old woman recently diagnosed with ovarian cancer. She had breast cancer at age twenty-five, which was successfully treated with a mastectomy. She feels that this second cancer is unfair and rages against it. She was a religious woman but now feels God is punishing her unfairly. She cannot resolve her anger and becomes progressively more depressed. In Kathy's case her diagnosis would be conflicted religious beliefs, anger at God, and depression as a result of her spiritual issue.

If there is an interprofessional team involved, then a board-certified chaplain, as the expert in spiritual care, provides the input and guidance as to the diagnosis and treatment plan with respect to spirituality. In situations where there is no interprofessional team, health care professionals identify the issues or make the diagnoses and develop the treatment plan. These clinicians are responsible for referring complex spiritual issues to a board-certified chaplain. For simple issues, such as a patient wanting to learn about yoga, meditation, or art or music therapy, the health care professional can make the appropriate referral or implement a course of action. For the more complex spiritual issues, referral to a board-certified chaplain or other spiritual care provider is critical. Use of decision-tree algorithms may facilitate development of a treatment or care plan. Figure 13 is an example of one such algorithm. In this algorithm clinicians first must recognize patient distress, then identify if the distress is physical, psychosocial and/or, spiritual and then develop an appropriate treatment plan. Table 7 lists potential spiritual concerns or diagnoses with key features from the clinical history and example statements patients may make. Table 8 lists other symptoms the patient may present with that could be a factor if a primary spiritual diagnosis is present. For example, a patient may exhibit gallows humor but actually have a existential or spiritual crisis. Once a spiritual diagnosis is identified the clinician then develops the appropriate assessment and plan.

FIGURE 13   Spiritual Diagnosis Decision Pathway

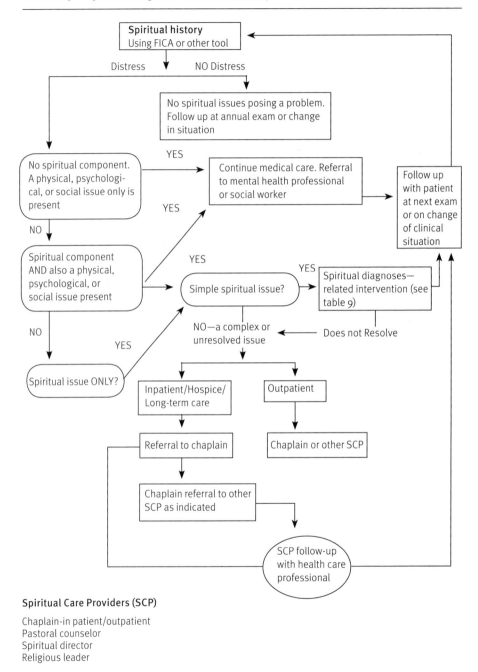

Spiritual Care Providers (SCP)

Chaplain-in patient/outpatient
Pastoral counselor
Spiritual director
Religious leader

(Puchalski et al., 2009)

TABLE 7 Spiritual Concerns or Diagnoses

Diagnoses (Primary)	Key Feature from History	Example Statements
Existential concerns	Lack of meaning Questions meaning about one's own existence Concern about afterlife Questions the meaning of suffering Seeks spiritual assistance	"My life is meaningless." "I feel useless."
Abandonment by God or others	Lack of love, loneliness Not being remembered No sense of relatedness	"God has abandoned me." "No one comes by anymore." "I am so alone."
Anger at God or others	Displaces anger toward religious representatives or others Inability to forgive	"Why would God take my child . . . it's not fair."
Concerns about relation- ship with diety	Desires closeness to God, deepening relationship	"I want to have a deeper relationship with God." "I want to understand my spirituality more."
Conflicted or challenged belief systems	Verbalizes inner conflicts or questions about beliefs of faith Conflicts between religious beliefs and recommended treatments Questions moral or ethical implications of therapeutic regimen Expresses concern with life/death or belief system	"I am not sure if God is with me anymore." "I question all that I used to hold as meaningful."
Despair/ hopelessness	Hopelessness about future health, life Despair as absolute hopelessness No hope for value in life	"Life is being cut short." "There is nothing left for me to live for."
Grief/loss	The feeling and process associated with the loss of a person, health, relationship	"I miss my loved one so much." "I wish I could run again."
Guilt/shame	Feeling that one has done something wrong or evil Feeling that one is bad or evil	"I do not deserve to die pain free."
Reconciliation	Need for forgiveness or reconciliation from self or others	"I need to be forgiven for what I did." "I would like my wife to forgive me."
Isolation	Separated from religious community or other community	"Since moving to the assisted living, I am not able to go to my church any-more." "I have moved and no longer can go to my usual 12-step meet-ing."
Religious specific	Ritual needs Unable to perform usual religious practices	"I just can't pray anymore."
Religious/ spiritual struggle	Loss of faith or meaning Religious or spiritual beliefs or com-munity not helping with coping	"What if all that I believe is not true?"

(Puchalski et al., 2009)

Identification of Spiritual Goals

During the clinical encounter, one can ask patients to develop an action plan with regard to their spirituality. In the FICA tool, the "A" refers to address or action, which can be included in the assessment of the treatment plan and can also be used as a question for the patient to assess his or her own spiritual journey or spiritual issue. For example, a patient may wish to build their skills in meditation or to be more intentional about a particular spiritual practice. Patients may also want to focus on reconciliation with others, God, or self. Reconciliation also calls for self-acceptance. Particularly for dying patients, a goal may be to achieve peacefulness in the face of impending death. In Kathy's case, spiritual counseling involved affirming her anger and her grief about being diagnosed with cancer. The chaplain helped Kathy reframe her situation and identify spiritual goals, which included finding acceptance and a sense of peace. Chaplains, pastoral counselors, and spiritual directors may be helpful as patients work on these spiritual issues.

Determining and Implementing the Appropriate Spiritual Intervention

Based on the diagnosis of spiritual distress, issues of resources of strength and the spiritual goals and appropriate interventions can be determined (see table 9). A patient may have concerns about meaning and purpose of his or her life and may benefit from spiritual counsel-

TABLE 8   Secondary Spiritual Diagnosis
(a primary spiritual diagnosis must be present to be considered spiritual)

Secondary
Behavior/mood alterations as evidenced by anger, crying, withdrawal, etc.
Pain
Feeling out of control
Uses gallows humor
Anger
Nightmares/sleep disturbances
Feelings of abandonment
Lack of trust

(NCCN Guidelines)

TABLE 9   Examples of Spiritual Health Interventions

Therapeutic Communication Techniques

1. Compassionate presence
2. Reflective listening, query about important life events
3. Support patient's sources of spiritual strength
4. Open-ended questions to illicit feelings
5. Inquiry about spiritual beliefs, values, and practices
6. Life review, listening to the patient's story
7. Continued presence and follow-up

Therapy

1. Referral to spiritual care provider as indicated
2. Guided visualization
3. Progressive relaxation
4. Breathing practice or contemplation
5. Meaning-oriented therapy
6. Use of storytelling
7. Dignity-conserving therapy

Self-Care

1. Massage
2. Reconciliation with self or others
3. Spiritual support groups
4. Meditation
5. Sacred/spiritual readings or rituals
6. Yoga, tai chi
7. Exercise
8. Art therapy (music, art, dance)
9. Journaling

---

ing. Thus a referral would be made to a spiritual care professional. Or a patient may be suffering from anxiety about death and fear about suffocating. A referral to a counselor and also teaching about breathing techniques may be helpful.

Continued compassionate presence is also part of the treatment plan. Simply being there for a patient and being open to his or her suffering can help resolve his or her spiritual crisis. Listening to a patient's story can also be healing or comforting. People often feel a sense of loneliness or abandonment when they are ill; having someone listen to them can assuage that sense of disconnection.

Board-certified chaplains will be integral to the initial interdisciplinary team evaluating the patient. Ideally chaplains will be involved in all parts of the assessment and development of the treatment plan. When chaplains are not available, clinicians need to find ways to consult with chaplains in developing the treatment or care plan. For recommendations about religious services and practices and for in-depth spiritual counseling, it is essential that chaplains lead the effort in this area.

The most prevalent contemporary model of chaplaincy is characterized by a commitment to meeting the spiritual needs of all patients and adherence to the principle of following the patient's lead. Well-educated, contemporary, board-certified chaplains are trained to respond to the needs of patients of all faiths and of no faith affiliation. Chaplains are prepared to meet the more specifically religious needs of patients as the patients' spiritual care demands it. A Muslim chaplain will most likely not be able to perform a Buddhist chant for a patient who requests it. Thus, if in following the patient's lead, it becomes clear that the patient needs services that can better be provided by a chaplain of the patient's denomination, or by clergy who are not on the hospital staff, there is an obligation to try to provide such services. Often, this will involve contacting the patient's own religious community on his or her behalf. In addition, where feasible, chaplains should have an extensive interfaith network of collaborating religious leaders willing to come to the hospital on an ad hoc basis to provide denominationally specific religious services.

If patients seek a deepening of their relationship with God or a higher power or a search for authenticity, a referral to a spiritual director may be appropriate. If a patient seeks counseling for mental health issues and has associated spiritual issues, a referral to a pastoral counselor may be warranted. Just as nonchaplain clinicians need to refer to chaplains for more specialized spiritual issues, chaplains refer to other clinicians for issues related to other disciplines or area of expertise. For example, a chaplain may identify depression or anxiety and would refer to a social worker, psychologist, or psychiatrist. Or a patient might benefit from meaning-oriented therapy or dignity-conserving methods.

Community clergy may need to be called in to see their congregants for religious-specific care. Or one can integrate a culturally based healer for patients who request that. In addition, mind-body professionals (e.g., massage therapists, Reiki practitioner) or artists (poets, musicians, art therapists) may be appropriate for some patients. Patients may also request yoga, tai chi, or dance as a way to express their spirituality.

Reevaluation and Follow-Up

The National Consensus Project Guidelines suggest that periodic reevaluation of the impact of spiritual/existential interventions and patient-family preferences be documented (NCP, 2009). Any time an assessment is made, whether related to pain, nutrition, or psychosocial/spiritual problems, it is of the utmost importance to follow up to determine the impact of the intervention and adjust the plan of care as needed (Fitchett, 2002).

Previous spiritual assessments should be revisited and acknowledgment made as to the relationships between the patient and providers. Evaluation should include consideration of the intervention applied, the change in disease state, the care transition, and the change in relationships. Reevaluation should occur as the disease progresses, at transitions to different types or levels of care, when care environments change, and when there is a change in care provider or change in personal relationships. As in all types of quality care, interventions and evaluations should be grounded in effective, open-ended, and empathetic communication (Lo et al., 2002). Use of a structured history and assessment tools can facilitate reevaluation efforts.

Documentation

Documenting the provision of spiritual care allows for communication about the intervention and the corresponding desired outcomes. Documentation should occur in the social history section of the intake history and physical of the patient's chart, as well as in the daily progress notes as applicable. Documentation of the intervention showing its value and effectiveness is key to quality care and provides knowledge to other members of the interprofessional team who share in the care of the patient. Health care professionals could consider documenting spiritual issues as part of a comprehensive biopsychosocial-spiritual

FIGURE 14   A Biopsychosocial-Spiritual Assessment and Plan

Case example: An eighty-year-old dying of end-stage colon cancer with well-controlled pain, some anxiety, unresolved family issues, and fear about dying. Assessment reveals:

Physical	Pain is well controlled; continue with current medication regimen. Nausea: still has episodes of nausea and vomiting, likely secondary to partial small bowel obstruction. Add octreotide to current regimen.
Emotional	Anxiety about dyspnea that may be associated with dying; anxiety affecting sleep at night. Referral to counselor for anxiety management and exploration of issues about dying. Add Ativan to pm medication regimen as needed.
Social	Patient has unresolved issues with family members as well as questions about funeral planning and costs—refer to social worker for possible family intervention as well as assistance with end-of-life planning.
Spiritual	Patient expresses fear about dying; seeks forgiveness from son for being a "distant dad." Referral to chaplain for spiritual counseling, consider forgiveness intervention, encourage discussion about fear of death; continue presence and support.

(Adapted from table in Puchalski, 2007)

FIGURE 15   A Biopsychosocial-Spiritual Discharge Plan

A sixty-five-year-old patient admitted for repair of hip fracture; surgery went well, without complications, also noted anxiety, separation from religious community. Has strong spiritual beliefs, good level of hope, strong family support. Spiritual goal includes deepening relationship with God. Expressed interest in learning meditation.

Physical	s/p ORIF for PT/OT
Emotional	Anxious about not being able to work; has panic attacks at night. Continue with alprazolam qhs; referral for counseling with social worker at rehab facility.
Social	Encourage family to visit at rehab facility.
Spiritual	Isolation from church community; goals to deepen relationship with God. Referral to chaplain at rehab facility; referral to spiritual director once discharged from rehab; provide list of meditation centers and teachers in patient's community.

(Puchalski et al., 2009)

assessment and plan. (See figures 14 and 15.) Sound clinical judgment should govern how much detail is provided in the documentation. Private content or information offered in confidence should be documented only to the extent that it directly affects the patient's clinical care of patients and is critical for other members of the interprofessional team to know.

There is a very little in the literature about documenting patients' spiritual beliefs and values, and poor recording of patients' religious and spiritual information is often reported. Chaplains often do not enter their assessments into the patient record. One study evaluating why nurses do not chart about spirituality cited the intrusiveness of questions about spirituality and a feeling that the assessment was not necessary (Swift et al., 2007). Yet given the evidence base supporting for assessing if spiritual distress or spiritual resources of strength, it's clear that training is necessary to help health care professionals recognize that asking about spirituality is not intrusive if done appropriately. An analogy can be made to the sexual history, now a routine part of a patient history. Initially, clinicians felt that asking a sexual history was intrusive. But with increasing training on how to ask as well as evidence that sexuality has health and quality of life implications, a sexual history has become a standard in clinical interviewing.

One other concern for some health care professionals is the amount of time needed to document patient information. Some health care professionals might feel that spirituality is "just one more thing I have to take time with." However, given practical tools, such as the FICA or HOPE, documentation can be brief yet informative. Time should not drive the standards of care; rather, tools should enable health care professionals to do what is appropriate in an efficient manner.

In documentation, it is important to document the essential aspects of the patient's spirituality. In many cases, only a patient's religious affiliation is entered into the database, but no detailed information about spirituality more broadly defined or how the spirituality is integrated into the treatment plan is available. A single checked item that the patient is "Baptist" or "Buddhist" provides little information or direction for comprehensive spiritual care. It is important to document what the spiritual belief, value, or practice is; how important that is in a person's life and what influence it has on how a patient understands health and illness and on their health care decision making; whether a patient has a spiritual community or group that provides support; and finally what the spiritual diagnosis is or the spiritual issues are in the plan with regard to the clinical situation.

My (Puchalski) father had surgery for colon cancer several years ago. In the preoperative area, the nurse asked if he had spiritual beliefs that would affect his stay at the hospital. He noted that he was Catholic and that what gave him greatest meaning was singing. The nurse asked him if he wanted to see a priest and he stated that was not necessary for him in the hospital. She also asked more about his singing and discovered that he was a former opera singer. She asked him to sing, which he did in the preoperative area, bringing great to joy to all of us present and comfort for himself, as music provides great solace to him. The nurse noted this in his chart. Once he was admitted to a floor postsurgery, the floor nurses encouraged him to use the incentive spirometer, which he did not find helpful. The nurses, reading about his singing in his chart, would then ask him to sing several times a day. His operatic training taught him to use his diaphragm; singing was therefore a great substitute for the incentive spirometer. It also brightened the lives of other patients and clinicians. One morning my father and his cardiologist sang a duet; a family member of a very seriously ill patient noted that sight of a patient and his doctor singing brought hope to his day. A spiritual history and the information in the chart can certainly impact the patient's care and overall care in significant ways.

Summary of Process

Once the clinician obtains the information from the history, he or she needs to decide how to integrate it into the treatment plan. The steps include making a diagnosis, identifying spiritual goals if appropriate, and determining and implementing the appropriate spiritual interventions. There are two possible pathways once a diagnosis is made: the simple and complex. For simple issues, such as a patient wanting to learn about yoga or meditation, the clinician can make the appropriate referral or course of action. For more complex spiritual and religious issues, referral to chaplains and other spiritual care professionals is critical.

A decision-tree algorithm (see figure 13) describes the path clinicians can follow in diagnosing and treating spiritual issues in patients. Tables 7 and 8 show possible presentations of symptoms of spiritual issues, including words and phrases patients may use. Table 9 shows the various interventions clinicians can offer. The figures and tables are shown above.

Documentation   Based on the biopsychosocial-spiritual model of care, one can view a treatment or care plan as grounded in this model. Thus, one would assess the physical, emotional, social, and spiritual aspects of patients; formulate a diagnosis or theory about how each of these dimensions affects the patient; and integrate this information into a treatment or care plan as appropriate. This plan would include input from the interdisciplinary team and would be updated on a regular basis with appropriate follow-up and reevaluation. An example of such an integrated plan is shown in figure 14. This same model can be applied to the discharge plan where each of these dimensions are included (see figure 15). This is one way to document spiritual concerns in a patient's chart.

The issue of time is sometimes raised as a barrier for providing compassionate care and for doing a patient-centered interview that includes a spiritual history. However, given the data as well as the ethical standards for providing patient-centered and culturally sensitive care, time should not take precedence over what is considered a good standard of care. In order to implement all these recommendations, however, our consensus group did suggest that effective and simple tools be utilized to assist clinicians in busy clinical practice settings.

Recommendations

1. Screen and assess every patient's spiritual symptoms, values, and beliefs and integrate them into the plan of care.
2. All trained health care professionals should do spiritual screening and history-taking. These caregivers should also identify any spiritual diagnoses and develop a plan of care. Detailed assessment and complex diagnosis and treatment are the purview of the board-certified chaplains working with the interprofessional team as the spiritual care experts.

3. Currently available diagnostic labels (e.g., National Comprehensive Cancer Network [NCCN] Distress Management guidelines, *Diagnostic and Statistical Manual* [*DSM*] code V62.89, NANDA nursing diagnoses) can be used, but further work is needed to develop more comprehensive diagnostic codes for spiritual problems.

4. Treatment plans should include but not be limited to:
   a. Referral to chaplains, spiritual directors, pastoral counselors, and other spiritual care providers, including clergy or faith-community healers for spiritual counseling
   b. Development of spiritual goals
   c. Meaning-oriented therapy
   d. Mind-body interventions
   e. Rituals, spiritual practices
   f. Contemplative interventions

5. Patients should be encouraged and supported in the expression of their spiritual needs and beliefs as they desire and this should be integrated into the treatment or care plan and reassessed periodically. Written material regarding spiritual care, including a description of the role of chaplains, should be made available to patients and families. Family and patient requests specifically related to desired rituals at any point in their care and particularly at the time of death should be honored.

6. Board-certified chaplains should function as spiritual care coordinators and help facilitate appropriate referrals to other spiritual care providers or spiritual therapies (e.g., meditation training) as needed.

7. Spiritual support resources from the patient's own spiritual/religious community should be noted in the chart.

8. Follow-up evaluations should be done regularly, especially when there is a change in status or level of care, or when a new diagnosis or prognosis is determined.

9. Treatment algorithms can be useful adjuncts to determine appropriate interventions.

10. The discharge plan of care should include all dimensions of care, including spiritual needs.

11. Spiritual care must extend to bereavement care. Palliative care programs should institute processes to ensure that systematic

bereavement support is provided. Referral to bereavement counselors or services should be available as appropriate for loved ones and families after the death of the patient. Structured bereavement assessment tools should be used to identify needs for support and those at greatest risk for complicated grief.

12. Health care professionals should establish procedures for contact with family or loved ones following the death of a patient. This may include sending condolences, attending funerals, holding memorial services, or other rituals to offer support to and connection with the family.

9 Interprofessional Considerations

Roles and Team Functioning

Theoretical, Empirical, and Philosophical Background

The Dynamics of Team Care

Excellent care at the end of life requires a team of caregivers, and this introduces the special ethical issues that arise in collective activity. Collaboration on interdisciplinary teams has become a central component in health care delivery systems (Abrahmson & Mizrahi, 2003; Dunevitz, 1997; Netting & Williams, 1996; Payne, 2000). No one clinician can possibly meet the requirement to be "comprehensive" in the sense of meeting the combined physical, psychosocial, spiritual, and personal needs of the dying person. While all have some responsibility for spiritual care, chaplains play a key role as the team members most directly responsible for spiritual care.

As The Joint Commission has asserted:

> The emerging prominent role of clinically trained, professional board-certified chaplains working with healthcare organizations in completing spiritual assessments, functioning as the "cultural broker," and leading cultural and spiritual sensitivity assessments for staff and physicians can be of great value. . . .
>
> Organizations that employ board-certified, professional chaplains are able to focus directly on the significance and incorporation of cultural, spiritual, and religious practices into the plan of care. . . .
>
> Organizations should actively involve professional healthcare pastoral care providers who are clinically trained and nationally board certified. (Tinoco, 2006, p. 76)

In the United States there has been no better example of how clinicians can work together as a team to provide such comprehensive care, including spiritual care, than the example provided by the hospice movement. Despite its advantages, however, team care raises a variety of issues.

First, one must decide how responsibilities are to be apportioned. Responsibility may reside in one team member or be assigned to each member relative to his or her function on the team, or there may be true collective responsibility in which each team member shares responsibility for the whole team's actions. These three approaches seem deeply intertwined, with no clear way to disentangle them entirely.

The physician writes the orders and is ultimately responsible for the patient's care. Nonetheless, nurses, chaplains, social workers, and psychologists are all professionals in their own right. They all have codes of ethics that make them responsible for the care they provide. No member of the team, not even the physician, can ask another member of the team to violate his or her professional ethics. Any member who cooperates in or fails to object to any harmful act is a moral accomplice. In that sense every team member shares in the collective responsibility of the whole team for the care provided.

One complicating ethical factor is the considerable overlap of roles and responsibilities in the spiritual care of the dying. For example, a psychologist, physician, and chaplain may all be addressing different aspects of a patient's anxieties about dying. All team members therefore have an obligation to apply their expertise humanely, sensitively, and compassionately, but they also have an obligation to communicate frequently and effectively to avoid redundancies and actions that might even be at cross-purposes.

Team dynamics can also raise ethical issues. In the interest of team harmony, members can become too compliant, or too eager to be seen as "good team players." They might lose the ability to see alternative ways of caring for patients or to challenge the plan put forth by the majority of the team's members. Others might be lulled by group dynamics into paying more attention to the "anguish of the caregiver" than to the anguish of the patient. Self-righteousness and self-pity are subtle tendencies in teams that attend dying and suffering patients and both should be eschewed. Finally, one must consider the proper exercise of the role of team leader. This is becoming less the role of a "captain" and more that of facilitator or convener. Patient and family members also have roles to play as members of the palliative care team.

An effective team has the following characteristics:

1. Respect of all team members for each other.
2. Effective and clear communication.
3. Openness to all members' suggestions and opinions.
4. Support for each teams' professional growth and development.
5. Values based in service to the patient and family.
6. Commitment of each team member to the delivery of compassionate high-quality patient- and family-centered care.

Good teamwork in palliative care involves constant evaluations of the care being delivered and a consistent reflection of the goals of care.

Community Spiritual Leaders

In addition to social workers, chaplains, physicians, and nurses, other spiritual professionals may participate as part of the larger team working with patients and families. These include community clergy, religious leaders, community elders, spiritual directors, pastoral counselors, and lay religious professionals. Community religious professionals can be a valuable resource for the palliative care team in providing care to patients and their loved ones. They may have known the patient and family over a long period of time and have a wide degree of access to them when they are out of the hospital, including visiting them at home. Many patients and families rely on their clergy for support at the end of life.

In building a relationship with a community religious professional, it is important for the team to determine that person's training. It is also important to determine that person's beliefs about how medical decisions should be made and how end-of-life care should proceed, especially with regard to the use of pain medication and life-sustaining treatments.

As already mentioned, training for religious professionals varies widely. In some communities, it is even considered unnecessary to have any education because God is the one who gives knowledge. Further, religious professionals who have graduate education may have no counseling training or exposure to the culture or processes of health care. Thus, until proven otherwise, religious professionals should be assumed to have knowledge of medical and palliative care issues at the same level as other lay people. There are various categories of religious or spiritual professionals that palliative care teams will potentially encounter in the community. These religioius or spiritual professionals vary considerably both within and across groups in training, credentials, and relationships to the palliative care client and their family caregivers.

Ordained Clergy, Religious Leaders, Community Elders Ordained clergy or other religious leaders or elders are generally the leaders of their religious communities. They are often looked to by the members of their congregation for guidance and counsel, including in regard to health care decisions. In some cases, congregants will cede decision-making authority about health care issues to these individuals who may or may not be available to the health care team. These decisions can include whether or not to take pain medicine and how to deal with advance directives. From a health care perspective, it is essential to note that the training of these clergy, religious leaders, and community elders varies widely. Some have graduate-level education in theology and clinical training in health care settings where they may even have been exposed to palliative care teams. In some congregations (e.g., the Community of Christ), church men and women clergy are called by church leaders and must accept the call personally. The call then needs to be approved by the congregation/district/mission center. After this process, study ensues. When that is complete, the ordination occurs. Others may not even have a college degree and their ordination was granted to them by their congregations solely on the basis of the determination that they had received a "call" from God, who is deemed to be the sole and only necessary source of their knowledge and authority. Others may not be officially ordained because their religious denominations do not ordain, but they function in a comparable role. The Church of the Latter Day Saints and some congregations of the Society of Friends (Quakers) would be examples of this. They can have vastly different ideas about their roles vis-à-vis their congregants and health care professionals. They may have little or no education in issues such as confidentiality. The question "By what authority is the person called?" is an important one, but it is also important to understand that in some congregations there are a number of distinct internal/external sources of authority.

Lay Religious Professionals   Many religious communities employ unordained people in various capacities that may bring them into contact with palliative care teams and other health care professionals. This can include religious educators, youth program directors, and music/ritual directors. While the main job responsibilities for these professionals do not generally involve ministry to the sick, this visitation is sometimes part of their responsibilities. They may also become involved in visitation by virtue of their contact with the patient or family through their regular job responsibilities. It would be unusual for anyone in this position to have any clinical training or training in ministry to the sick, including end-of-life care. While these are spiritual care professionals, they are generally not given the same authority as clergy, religious leaders, or community elders by congregants. An exception might be when the congregation is without a clergyman or is in a group that does not ordain, as mentioned above.

It is important to note that some congregations employ a professional either as a regular member of the staff or as a consultant to run bereavement programs. Again, while the training of these counselors varies, some are fully trained bereavement professionals who can be of significant assistance to a palliative care team. They also may run programs in their congregations open to nonmembers of that congregation.

Stephen Ministry is a lay Christian program that provides training for the laity to be caring ministers in a congregation, or lay spiritual care volunteers. Stephen Ministers provide one-to-one care for the bereaved, hospitalized, terminally ill, separated, divorced, unemployed, and others facing a crisis or life challenge.

Pastoral Counselor   Certified pastoral counselors are a distinct branch of the pastoral care profession. They are sometimes called "pastoral psychotherapists," which is a useful descriptor. Most are ordained, but ordination is not required. While health care chaplains are trained to do short-term or crisis counseling in acute care settings, pastoral counselors are trained to do longer-term therapy. The American Association of Pastoral Counselors (AAPC, n.d.) states that "pastoral counseling moves beyond the support or encouragement a religious community can offer, by providing psychologically sound therapy that weaves in the religious and spiritual dimension." To be certified by the AAPC, a counselor must have at least 375 hours of pastoral counseling together with 125 hours of supervision by a certified counselor. Many pastoral counselors also have advanced degrees in clinical psychology or social work. A major caution is that pastoral counselors are not licensed in most states. Therefore, anyone can legally call him- or herself a pastoral counselor without regard to credentials or training. It is recommended that referrals only be made to counselors certified by the AAPC and so listed on their website (www.aapc.org). Pastoral counselors can be on the staff of congregations but can also have solo or group practices normally called pastoral counseling centers. While like most counselors they have differing subspecialties, they generally have experience with grief and bereavement issues and work with families.

Spiritual Directors   A spiritual director accompanies people on a spiritual journey. The art of spiritual direction exists in a context that emphasizes growing closer to God (or the holy or a higher power). Spiritual directors invite their directees to forge a deeper relationship with the spiritual aspect of being human. Spiritual directors are not counselors; rather, they are trained to be a companion to the other in his or her spiritual journey, assisting with noticing and discerning God's or the divine's presence and movement.

Since 2000 there has been increased interest in the practice of spiritual direction, both from people feeling called to be spiritual directors and from those seeking direction. The growth in the number of directors has also necessitated an increased need to train those who supervise them. Spiritual directors, who have years of experience in supervision, explore a wide variety of issues with their trainees, including gender and sexuality, ethical dilemmas, working with diverse racial ethnic constituents, working with the differently disabled, the parameters of supervision, the supervision of beginning directors, and more.

Certificates in spiritual direction are created by some institutions (e.g., Washington Theological Union) to support and further the development of those called to the ministry of spiritual direction. The core requirements include a historical study of spiritual direction and its theological underpinnings, related spiritual themes, and a supervised exploration of the process and skills of spiritual direction. The core is complemented by other courses related to spirituality and other electives of interest. Each candidate is expected to receive regular spiritual direction and maintain a personal spiritual practice that attends to his or her relationship with God/the sacred and nurtures a contemplative stance toward life and ministry. Completion of the certificate indicates mastery of the course content and advanced skills in accompanying others along their spiritual path. Continued peer or individual supervision is recommended and expected beyond the completion of the program.

Theological Perspective

Patients, family members, and religious professionals alike tend to have theological perspectives that color how they view palliative care and medical decisions. The salient piece of the theological perspective for this discussion is the issue of authority in decision making. For purposes of discussion, the two important groups in religion can be called "negotiators" and "traditional." For negotiators, the authority to make decisions rests jointly with the patient and his or her religious authorities such as clergy, or religious leaders, and sacred texts. Thus, the patient negotiates decisions. Most health care providers are negotiators in this sense. For those that are traditional, all authority is external. That is, sacred text or the clergy or religious leaders who interpret those texts are viewed as having complete authority to make decisions. It is important for health care providers to understand when they are dealing with a traditional religious professional because they may not be open to discussion about particular circumstances. They expect to give their congregant the answer and that the congregant will generally follow it. If at all possible, religious professionals in this group should be dealt with by a professional chaplain with experience in this kind of negotiation. Virtually all religious "rules" have exceptions or there are recognized extenuating circumstances. Being successful in this kind of negotiation often entails understanding where these sometimes arcane exceptions lie and being able to discuss these with the clergy or religious leader in the context of what is happening to the patient.

Communication among health care professionals, including spiritual care professionals, is a critical element of interdisciplinary care. In the hospice, hospital, or long-term care setting, interdisciplinary rounds may be the way most communication occurs. In addition, notes in the patient record are essential to communicate spiritual concerns. It is critical that communication occur in ways in which the patient's spiritual issues can be fully explored and integrated. One challenging situation in clinical settings is how clergy, religious leaders, and other spiritual care professionals not on the hospital staff communicate with hospital health care professionals. The HIPAA (Health Insurance Portability and Accountability Act of 1966) guidelines concerning confidentiality have created some barriers to recognition of nonhospital clergy and religious leaders as members of the health care team, thus limiting access to patient information. Communication also has implications for patient confidentiality. Some of the issues that affect the communication between spiritual care professions and other clinicians include time and the hectic pace of the current health care system, lack of a fully functional interdisciplinary team, and lack of understanding on the part of clinicians about the role of chaplains and other spiritual care professionals.

Clinical settings need to hold all clinicians and chaplains accountable for communicating with each other about patient care. They should outline specific strategies for sharing patient clinical information with each other. For example, a hospital should integrate chaplain notes into the patient medical database and charts in the section where clinicians chart. There should be a mechanism for spiritual care professionals who are not part of the hospital staff to communicate their concerns about patients to the hospital chaplain who in turn can relate the information to the other clinicians involved. Chaplains can serve as spiritual care coordinators. Finally, the pace and business of the hospital environment should not be an issue if communication issues can be streamlined, as in the chart, in brief meetings, or through electronic messaging or "tasking" of colleagues. In addition, spiritual history tools, such as the FICA tool, take only one to two minutes and can be done in a time-efficient manner. Also, experienced clinicians know how to utilize all parts of the clinical visit to obtain needed clinical information.

For example, while doing a physical exam, clinicians continue to have conversations about a variety of issues. Finally, compassion is intention dependent, not time dependent. Thus, a clinician can be fully present, attentive, and compassionate in any encounter with the patient, regardless of how long that encounter is. By holding all health care professionals accountable for spiritual care, communication between clinicians and spiritual care professionals should improve.

The notion of spiritual care provided by a team of caregivers raises specific questions about confidentiality. Patients might be inclined to divulge different kinds of personal information to different members of the team for differing purposes and reasons. This raises ethical tensions when one considers the important duty of sharing of information to facilitate good communication and delivery of comprehensive care by a team. Judgments about what information to share and when and how to do so will always require clinical judgment, and no simple rules can be provided. The safest and wisest rule, however, will always be to secure the patient's permission, when feasible, before sharing privately communicated information with other members of the team. A physician, for instance, after discovering that a patient is in the throes of a significant spiritual crisis, might say to the patient, "Thank you for trusting me enough to share what you're going through. I think we need to try to find a way to help you. As you know, however, I'm not a chaplain. With your permission I'd like to share a little about what we've discussed with Chaplain Smith, who is part of our team. She's the expert on these matters. I'll ask her to drop by later and pick up on these important matters with you." Likewise, a chaplain might say, "This has been a very important discussion and it has certainly helped me to understand more about why you don't want to have the CT scan. Would you mind if I shared some of what you've said with Dr. Smith? She is really concerned about you, but I don't think she has fully understood how much you consider this a matter between you and God. I think it would really help her to work with you if I could explain this a little. Does that sound like a good plan?"

These same moral considerations should guide the writing of notes. We fully endorse and encourage chaplains to write notes in the chart, since this facilitates team communication and coordinated care for patients as whole persons. However, chaplains must exercise prudence in doing so. Merely noting that one visited the patient seems inadequate; however, writing long notes detailing intimate details of a patient's spiritual journey that might not be very relevant to the care delivered by other members of the team needlessly puts the privacy of patients at risk for unclear gains. As in verbal communication, securing the permission of the patient to share the information and assuring that it is for a clinically relevant reason seem good ethical rules of thumb to guide the writing of notes by chaplains.

Health care professionals have training and guidelines on confidentiality. These are specified in HIPAA and ethical and professional guidelines. Community religious professionals also have a range of conceptions of confidentiality. Those who have had clinical training in a hospital probably understand the normal rules for health care fairly well. However, there is a widespread understanding among many clergy, religious leaders, and laity that all communication among clergy, religious leaders, and their congregants is confidential. More importantly, many lay people also understand communication with clergy to be subject to a much higher standard of confidentiality than communication with other professionals. This understanding reflects the Christian understanding of the "seal of the confessional" that prescribes that all communication among clergy, religious leaders, and penitent is sealed and cannot be divulged. Over time, many religious people have lost the distinction between confession and other kinds of communication with clergy and religious leaders. Even within the hospital, it is not uncommon for patients to assume that communication with a chaplain is held to a different standard of confidentiality than communication with other health care professionals.

Many community clergy and religious leaders between them have a right to health care information about congregants. This tradition has been interrupted by HIPAA, but many clergy and religious leaders still believe that they should be given information on congregants when they ask. Seeking consent from the patient and family is critical to help resolve both of these dilemmas. Often patients want their clergy or religious leaders to understand their medical situation and are glad to give consent for that sharing. Likewise, the trained clergy or religious leader should be able and willing to ask congregants if information can be shared with the health care team and explain the reasons.

In general because of the HIPPA concerns, it is not feasible for clergy to obtain information on patients or to document notes in patients' charts. It is recommended that clergy work through the pastoral or spiritual care office and utilize chaplains as a spiritual care manager, where chaplains can help facilitate clergy visits and information sharing in the hospital or long-term care settings.

Practice Principles

The first step in valuing a health care system as a spiritual community is to develop greater awareness of one's own spiritual self. Walking a spiritual path helps us identify our own spiritual capacities for nurturing and our vulnerabilities (Nelson-Becker, 2008). Vulnerability is a call to attention that in a weak place we have a task to accomplish. Awareness brought to vulnerable places can lead to reflection and self-work that ultimately can create strength. Our spiritual journey becomes the context through which we filter our understanding of patients, the stories they share, and our relationships with other members in this healing community.

The second step in working with members of health care systems is to cocreate healing environments. This involves recognition that spiritual presence is a key aspect of the healing capacity of groups. It would be wise for groups to have an explicit discussion about their spiritual and nonspiritual viewpoints, understanding that the convergence in knowledge and acceptance of diverse worldviews will create greater ability in teams to meet explicit and implicit needs of patients and family members (Milliken & Martins, 1996). Where a member of a team has an expressly nonspiritual worldview, it is important for the team to recognize the value this has for the team: it keeps team members aware of their own biases and values and ultimately widens the group capacity to work with diverse patients and situations.

The third step is to view the health care systems as intentional spiritual communities where members respect each other's diversity of beliefs and values and honor each other's dignity. Beginning with each other, they can be open to sharing and hearing the everyday challenges that lead to deep learning. So much of our lives remain undisclosed and untold. Team members can learn from each other in the process of sharing appropriately about the challenges team members encounter in their professional work. This is not to suggest that team members become therapists for each other. That action would add undue burden. However, it is in the spiritual connections we make with others that we find sustaining grace. Who among us has not been strengthened by the heroic behavior of our patients and their families? Courageously reaching out to affirm others in their vulnerabilities, hopes, and dreams is a spiritual gift. It is a model toward which health care systems can and should move.

The fourth step is to recognize that while all members are equal as human beings, professionally there are differing skills, training, and certifications. Recognition of and respecting these differences is crucial to ethical team communication. Thus, the chaplain may identify physical issues with patients but would refer those issues to the physician and nurse. The physicians and nurses may do a spiritual history but would refer to the chaplain for more in-depth spiritual counseling. Figure 16 provides a guide for interdisciplinary collaborative spiritual care (GWish, 2008).

Outpatient Setting

The lack of a full interdisciplinary team in the outpatient setting presents a challenge. This situation is likely to be particularly difficult for the delivery of spiritual care because there are no generally accepted guidelines or practices in this arena. In the outpatient setting, it is easy to assume that any patient or family member who desires spiritual care or who would find it useful has spiritual or religious resources and a community to provide for that need. However, Balboni et al. (2007) found that in their study of spiritual needs 49 percent of patients with advanced cancer did not have their religious and spiritual needs met by their faith community. This is because patients are not routinely asked about their spirituality and do not have their spiritual issues integrated into treatment care plans. In their faith communities it may be that the focus is on religious-specific issues, such as rituals, but not on spiritual issues such as despair or meaninglessness. Mr. Wong was an elderly man from China who was being cared for in an outpatient setting for end-stage COPD. His doctors assumed he was Buddhist, as that was written in his chart. He continued to be despondent despite the addition of antidepressants to his treatment plan. On one visit,

FIGURE 16   A Guide for Interdisciplinary Collaborative Spiritual Care

Preamble: The application of the Guide for Interdisciplinary Collaborative Spiritual Care is to promote meaningful, compassionate care that addresses the spiritual dimension of an individual. The spiritual dimension is an essential part of the individual's personal striving for health, wholeness, and meaning of life. One's definition of spirituality is very individualized and may or may not include a religious preference.

This guide serves as a guide for how health care professionals can honor, integrate, and bring to light the spiritual underpinnings of collective ethical codes for a mutual goal of achieving the highest possible level of health and healing for all.

Collaborators: Patients, families, and a variety of health and spiritual care professionals, such as health care chaplains/clergypersons/spiritual and religious leaders, culturally based healers, mind-body practitioners, nurses, physicians, psychologists, public health researchers and social workers, community health educators.

Shared Values: Autonomy, compassion, competence, confidentiality, courage, dignity, equality, generosity, humility, integrity, justice, respect, reverence, trust, and worth

Guiding Documents: American Psychological Association's Code of Ethics, American Medical Association's Principles of Medical Ethics, American Nursing Association's Code of Ethics, Association of Professional Chaplains' Code of Ethics, National Association of Catholic Chaplains' Code of Ethics, National Association of Social Workers' Code of Ethics, Public Health Leadership Society's Principles of the Ethical Practice of Public Health, and Unified Code of Ethics for Healers.

This code of ethics for professional health care providers' collective professional organizations affirms the following for health care professionals in the provision of spiritual care:

Provide competent and compassionate spiritual care.

Recognize spirituality as an integral component to the human experience of illness, healing, and health.

Perform spiritual inquiry in a patient-centered, confidential, and respectful manner.

Elicit the patient's ongoing spiritual concerns/issues/needs.

Be sensitive to the ways in which a patient describes spiritual beliefs, practices, values, meaning, and relationships.

Patient autonomy shall be respected as the patient chooses to address spirituality; or not to address spirituality.

Practice spiritual self-care as a provider of spiritual care.

Collaborate with qualified interdisciplinary professionals.

Work in partnership in the study, application, and advancement of scientific knowledge regarding spirituality and health care.

Perform only those services for which qualified; observe all laws; and uphold the dignity and honor of one's profession.

(Gwish, 2008)

a resident physician asked a spiritual history. He found out that Mr. Wong had converted to Catholicism in his country illegally and was afraid to have that documented on his charts. He wanted the sacrament of the anointing of the sick (formerly called "last rites") and was "depressed," as he felt he would die without that sacrament. He also felt disconnected from his family because he had never shared his conversion and wanted to reconcile with them.

Asking a spiritual history is an important way to uncover what is important to the patient. In Mr. Wong's case, a chaplain referral would have helped, but there was no chaplain in the outpatient setting. Mr. Wong was connected with a priest who did perform "last rites," but did not explore some of the other spiritual issues the patient presented. The team made a referral to hospice and the patient was seen by a chaplain at the home visits. It is often the case that the patients and caregivers in outpatient settings will not have a regular chaplain available to them. It would not be uncommon for an outpatient clinic to have hundreds of patients seen each day in the outpatient setting, yet have no chaplain available. The Joint Commission (2008) only requires that accredited institutions "accommodate" spiritual and religious needs and does not require that a chaplain or spiritual care provider of any kind be available. Many hospitals and long-term care facilities provide for these needs only by calling community clergy or religious leaders on an ad hoc, volunteer basis. More care is being shifted to the outpatient setting as a result of economics and the aging of the population. This shift of care has an impact on the challenge of providing spiritual care to patients and families. Therefore, models need to be developed where chaplaincy needs to be available in the outpatient setting.

Recommendations

1. Policies about effective and appropriate communication channels between health care professionals and spiritual care professionals in a variety of health care settings are needed.
2. Policies should be developed by clinical sites to facilitate networking, communication, and coordination among spiritual care providers. Board-certified chaplains can function as spiritual care coordinators to facilitate this communication.

3. Health care professionals should work to create healing environments in their workplace.
4. Respect for the dignity of all health care professionals should be reflected in policies (e.g., a hospital code of ethics could include respect for fellow workers and treating all with compassion).
5. Spiritual care providers should document their assessment of patient needs in the patient record and contribute to the treatment plans as appropriate as part of interprofessional communication and collaboration.
6. Given the significant shift in health care to outpatient settings, there is a need for board-certified chaplains in these areas. Initial screening and some treatment of spiritual issues may be done by health care professionals such as physicians, counselors, parish nurses, and social workers. More complex spiritual issues need to be attended to by a board-certified chaplain or equivalently prepared spiritual care provider.
7. Activities and programs to enhance team spirit and system-wide compassion and respect can be introduced into the workplace. These can include retreats, opportunities for reflection, team-building experiences, and service recognition awards for compassionate care.

Theoretical, Empirical, and Philosophical Background and Practice Principles

Over the last decade there has been a significant increase in formal education in spirituality in health in the nonchaplain professions. Over 85 percent of medical and osteopathic schools have topics related to spirituality integrated into the curriculum. Nursing has integrated spirituality into the essentials of baccalaureate training. Social work programs have spirituality integrated into their undergraduate and master's program. The Marie Curie Cancer Care Center (n.d.) in the United Kingdom has developed a set of competencies for health care providers for spiritual care.

Health care professionals are recognizing that there are inadequacies in the health care system in terms of care of the dying. The American College of Physicians convened an end-of-life consensus panel that concluded that physicians should extend their care for those with serious medical illness by attentiveness to psychosocial, existential, or spiritual suffering (Lo et. al., 1999). Other national organizations including the American Association of Colleges of Nursing (2008) have also supported the inclusion of spirituality in the clinical setting. The Joint Commission policy states: "Pastoral counseling and other spiritual services are often an integral part of the patient's daily life. When requested, the hospital provides, or provides for, pastoral counseling services."

Medicine

Interest in spirituality among medical educators has been growing exponentially. Medical schools are now teaching courses in end-of-life care and in spirituality and medicine. Only one school had a formal course in spirituality and medicine in 1992. Today more than one hundred medical schools are teaching such courses (Puchalski & Larson, 1998; Puchalski, 2006b). A key element of these courses addresses listening to what is important to patients, respecting spiritual beliefs, and being able to communicate effectively with them about their spiritual belief and preferences at the end of life and across the life span.

The Association of American Medical Colleges (AAMC) developed the Medical School Objectives Project (MSOP), and Report I (AAMC, 1998) supports the need for physicians to "seek to understand the meaning of the patients' stories in the context of the patients' and family and cultural values" (p. 4). In 1999, with support from the John Templeton Foundation, a consensus conference with AAMC was convened to determine learning objectives and methods of teaching courses on spirituality, cultural issues, and end-of-life care. The findings of the conference were published as Report III. This report included a clinically relevant definition of spirituality:

> Spirituality is recognized as a factor that contributes to health in many persons. The concept of spirituality is found in all cultures and societies. It is expressed in an individual's search for ultimate meaning through participation in religion and/or belief in God, family, naturalism, rationalism, humanism, and the arts. All of these factors can influence how patients and health care professionals perceive health and illness and how they interact with one another. (p. 25)

The outcome goals stated in MSOP Report III are that students will:

- Be aware that spirituality, as well as cultural beliefs and practices, are important elements of the health and well-being of many patients.
- Be aware of the need to incorporate awareness of spirituality, and cultural beliefs and practices, into the care of patients in a variety of clinical contexts.
- Recognize that their own spirituality, and cultural beliefs and practices, might affect the ways they relate to, and provide care to, patients.
- Be aware of the range of end-of-life care issues and when such issues have or should become a focus for the patient, the patient's family, and members of the health care team involved in the care of the patient.

- Be aware of the need to respond not only to the physical needs that occur at the end of life, but also to the emotional, sociocultural, and spiritual needs that occur.

There has also been an increase in training in spirituality and health in residency programs, either as stand-alone topics or integrated into training in palliative and end-of-life care (Weissman et al., 2001). These are all very positive signs pointing to increased training for physicians in spiritual care. Ongoing support of these efforts is needed. There has been a significant increase in palliative medicine education in medical schools and residencies (Weissman et al., 2007). Palliative care physicians are certified through the American College of Physicians. Their certification requirements include the integration of the spiritual dimension of patients in their care.

Nursing

Nursing schools are currently interested in developing more spiritual care content in their baccalaureate courses. In 2008 the Essentials of Baccalaureate Education for Professional Nursing Practice (AACN, 2008) was updated to include competencies in spirituality into all of the nine essentials. The End-of-Life Nursing Education Consortium (ELNEC) program is a national continuing education program for nurses that addresses spirituality as a dimension of palliative care. The ELNEC project has trained over ten thousand nurses in the United States representing all fifty states and more than sixty countries (ELNEC, 2009). Nurses have also been leaders in teaching spiritual care at both undergraduate and graduate levels and in implementing spiritual care in continuing education.

Faith in community nursing has an extensive curriculum on integration of spirituality into care of patients. A parish nurse is a registered nurse with additional training who serves members of the congregation and people in the community as well. The role of a parish nurse is to be an educator, health counselor, communication link, organizer of support groups, and resource.

Social Work

Quality palliative care is best delivered in a collaborative environment by skilled medical, nursing, and psycho-oncology professionals integrating a biopsychosocial-spiritual model. The complex interplay of physical, psychological, social, spiritual, existential, medical, financial, and social burdens experienced by those diagnosed with cancer make a team approach imperative. The delivery of quality palliative care requires competent and compassionate professionals who have the education and experience to address the complex concerns of cancer patients and their families.

The National Consensus Project Guidelines (2009) encourage palliative care professionals to integrate patient and family spiritual and cultural concerns into their delivery of care. Similarly, the National Comprehensive Cancer Network (NCCN, 2008) has annually updated algorithms for distress management and palliative care (NCCN, 2009) that have been adopted in many cancer institutions and that include spiritual and existential patient concerns. Meeting these recommendations requires a cadre of skilled practitioners who recognize the tremendous religious, spiritual, ethnic, and cultural diversity in cancer populations and the importance these variables play in serious illness, and who can work effectively together to promote patient care.

Despite growing recognition of the deficits in the delivery of quality psychosocial-spiritual care, there are few national interdisciplinary training programs for health care professionals. Patient and family psychosocial and spiritual concerns continue to be unreliably and inconsistently addressed. One program incorporates the National Consensus Project Guidelines and a quality-of-life model in its curriculum. The course seeks to ignite a commitment to transform the delivery of palliative care by providing psycho-oncology professionals with leadership skills, mentorship, and support. The premise of this project is that more effective team functioning, collaboration, and advocacy are necessary to systemically improve the delivery of palliative, end-of-life, and bereavement care. Nine major topic areas are included in the curriculum: the moral imperative to improve palliative care; personal death awareness; ethical obligations of psycho-oncology professionals; physical aspects; psychosocial aspects; spiritual aspects; advocacy; the role of the transdisciplinary team; and bringing together passion, knowledge, and action for effective change. Personal death-awareness exercises and legacy-building strategies provide practitioners with an opportunity to personalize their commitment to improve the delivery of quality palliative and bereavement care within their scope of influence. Extensive pre- and postcourse evaluations and six- and twelve-month follow-up surveys support the efficacy of the educational design (NCP, 2009; Otis-Green et al., 2009).

The Advanced Certified Hospice and Palliative Social Worker (ACHP-SW) credential was developed jointly by the National Hospice and Palliative Care Organization (NHPCO) and the National Association of Social Workers (NASW) in 2008. This credential was designed by social work leaders in hospice and palliative care for social workers who meet standards of excellence. This new national credential was tailored to recognize the knowledge, skills, and abilities necessary for social workers in hospice and palliative care settings. The credential developed in response to the Centers for Medicare and Medicaid Services requirement that hospices employ professional social workers and The Joint Commission recommendation that social workers be included on professional teams.

Chaplaincy

Chaplains are identified leaders (whether ordained, commissioned, or otherwise set aside by their religious tradition community) who have acquired an extended education in pastoral or spiritual care. All board-certified chaplains have at least 1,600 hours of clinical pastoral education (CPE). CPE is an interfaith professional education for ministry. It brings theological students and ministers of all faiths (pastors, priests, rabbis, imams, and others) into supervised encounters with persons in crisis. Out of an intense involvement with persons in need and the feedback from peers and teachers, students develop new awareness of themselves as persons and the needs of those to whom they minister. From theological reflection on specific human situations, they gain a new understanding of ministry. Within the interdisciplinary team process of helping people, they develop skills in interpersonal and interprofessional relationships.

CPE units are accredited in hospital institutions through their certifying organizations. In North America, chaplains are certified by at least one of the national organizations that are recognized by The Joint Commission for Accreditation of Pastoral Services. This includes Association of Professional Chaplains (approximately 3,700 members), The

Canadian Association for Pastoral Practice and Education (approximately 1,000 members), National Association of Catholic Chaplains (approximately 4,000 members), and the National Association of Jewish Chaplains (approximately 400 members).

Clinical work in the hospital setting, didactic group process, individual supervision, and peer review create the environment for the chaplain's spiritual and psychological growth. Guidance is given before and after hospital visits with patients and families. The supervisor has been trained through many years of self-introspection and therapy, group dynamics, and theological reflections to enhance the chaplain's awareness and effectiveness. All board-certified chaplains adhere to a code of professional ethics for health care chaplains and continue to complete annual education requirements. Confidentiality and sensitivity to multicultural and multifaith realities are core to the spiritual engagement of chaplain and patient. This specialized education enables chaplains to mobilize their spiritual resources so that their pastoral encounters and interventions fully address the needs of their hospital constituency. Appendix E summarizes the Spiritual Care Collaborative (2007) recommendations for training and certification of chaplains.

Community Spiritual Care Professionals

Community religious professionals often lack the training to be full partners in the palliative care enterprise. However, there are numerous opportunities to provide training for these professionals to help them better serve their constituents and be more productive partners for the palliative care team. Clergy or religious leaders understand that caring for those at the end of life is part of their role. They are often very receptive to training regarding end-of-life and palliative care issues. Clergy and religious leaders and their congregations are also receptive to members of the palliative care team providing education to their congregations. There are several programs that provide continuing education for clergy and religious leaders in spirituality and health or in end-of-life care. One of the first of such programs was Compassion Sabbath, a program on end-of-life care for clergy started by the Center for Bioethics in Kansas (http://www.practicalbioethics .org/cpb.aspx?pgID=866). The George Washington Institute for Spirituality and Health at George Washington University has a Summer Institute in Spirituality and Health Care, which offers training for all health care professionals, including clergy and other religious and spiritual leaders in spirituality and health (www.gwish.org). The Duke Institute on Care at the End of Life (www.iceol.duke.edu) offers many seminars and conferences for clergy and other religious leaders. Finally, Hospice Foundation of America sponsors an audio series on end-of-life issues for clergy and religious leaders called "Clergy to Clergy" (www.hospicefoundation.org).

Psychology

The formal involvement of psychology in palliative and end-of-life care is relatively recent compared to other disciplines focused on the psychosocial need of patients with advanced illness and their caregivers. Therefore, many psychologists also may not have received sufficient training in palliative and end-of life care. However, the American Psychological Association (APA) has recognized the need for the involvement of psychologists in end-of-life care and formal opportunities are beginning to emerge. The Veterans Administration has funded six interprofessional postdoctoral fellowships for psychologists in palliative care and hospice. The APA-approved fellowship is a one-year training program in which psychology fellows join the interdisciplinary palliative care team, including other fellows in social work, palliative medicine, nursing, and chaplaincy. The fellowships are designed to maximize expertise in psychological aspects of end-of life care and knowledge and treatment of common end-of-life psychiatric syndromes, including depression, anxiety, delirium, post-traumatic stress disorder, anticipatory grief, substance abuse, and sleep disorders. Fellows learn to identify and address spiritual and religious concerns related to chronic illness and death and dying and collaborate with other disciplines including physicians, chaplains, social workers, and nurses. Through formal didactic instruction and work with chaplain fellows and faculty members, psychology fellows develop an understanding of the spiritual and religious aspects of advanced illness and end-of-life care and learn how to possibly integrate exploration of these aspects in their work with patients.

Additionally, the APA recently funded a project for the development of a continuing education curriculum focused on end-of-life care for psychologists. This is a program of ten interactive training modules with course content based on current practice and research. To promote more understanding of the significance of religion and spirituality, it describes approaches to conducting spiritual screening for patients near the end of life and explains the coping mechanisms as well as conflicts associated with spirituality and religion near the end of life.

Physician Assistants

Physician assistant (PA) education, like medical school education, has had an increase in the number of courses in palliative care and spirituality and health. Paramount in PA education is recognition, respect, and a nonjudgmental attitude for diversity—spiritual, cultural, and ethnic across all of care, regardless of clinical situation. There are many PA programs that now integrate spirituality into the curriculum as well as sessions on end-of-life care, breaking bad news, and pain and symptom management in advanced illness.

Accreditation for PA programs comes via the Accreditation Review Commission on Education for the Physician Assistant, Inc. The standards listed in the Accreditation Review Commission are the minimum requirements needed to certify a program, and have been endorsed by the American College of Physicians, American College of Surgeons, and the American Medical Association, among others. Mandated content includes instruction on end-of-life care, counseling patients and families coping with illness and injury, exploration of end-of-life issues, and respect for the diversity of patients, including beliefs and values.

Recommendations

1. All members of the palliative care team should be trained in spiritual care. This training should be required as part of continuing education for all clinicians. At a minimum, content of these educational programs should include:

    a. All team members should have training in spiritual care commensurate with their scope of practice in regard to the spiritual care model. Health care professionals should be trained in doing a spiritual screening or history.

b. Health care professionals who are involved in diagnosis and treatment of clinical problems, and who are involved in referring patients to specialists or resources should know the basics of spiritual diagnosis and treatment.

c. All team members should have knowledge of the options for addressing patients' spirituality, including spiritual resources and information.

d. Health care professionals should be trained in the tenets of different faiths and in different cultures in order to provide culturally and spiritually competent care.

e. As part of their training in cultural competency, all team members should have a broad minimum level of training in the spiritual/religious values and beliefs that may influence patient and family decisions regarding life-sustaining treatment and palliative care.

f. All team members should be aware of the training and differences in spiritual care providers and know when to refer to each.

g. All team members should have training in compassionate presence and active listening, and practice these competencies as part of the interprofessional team.

2. Team members should have training in self-care, self-reflection, contemplative practice, and spiritual self-care.

3. Health care systems should offer time for professional development of staff with regard to spiritual care and develop accountability measures in spiritual care for the interprofessional team.

4. Board-certified chaplains can provide spiritual care education and support for the interprofessional team members.

5. Clinical sites should offer education for community clergy members and spiritual care providers about end-of-life care, procedures in health care facilities, palliative care, patient confidentiality, self-care, and how to support health care professionals in their professional development. Education for seminary students regarding end-of-life care can be facilitated by collaborating with seminary accreditation organizations.

6. Development of chaplain certification and training in palliative care is needed.

7. Profession-specific (e.g., medicine, nursing, social work, psychology) competencies and training in spiritual care should be developed.
8. Spiritual education models should be interdisciplinary. Examples of educational programs that could be utilized include those from the Marie Curie Cancer Center in London and the George Washington Institute for Spirituality and Health in Washington, DC.

11 Personal and Professional Development

Theoretical, Empirical, and Philosophical Background

Spiritual care emphasizes the importance of the relationship between two people (Puchalski, 2008). The clinician may be the professional expert in most of the encounter, but he or she is still a human being. By relating from our humanness, we can help form deeper and more meaningful connections with our patients. What this requires is awareness of the clinician's own values, beliefs, and attitudes, particularly toward his or her own mortality. The stress of working with seriously ill and dying patients can be facilitated by attentiveness to one's own spiritual and values framework. Many physicians and nurses speak of their own spiritual practices and how those practices help them deliver good spiritual care and, in fact, good medical care. One study also showed that daily spiritual experiences might help mitigate burn-out in the workplace (Holland & Neimeyer, 2005).

Professional Development and Spiritual Formation

In an address to the American Medical Association in 1957 (Sulmasy, 2006), Abraham Heschel, the late, great twentieth-century Jewish philosopher and theologian, told the assembled delegates, "To heal a person, one must first be a person" (p. 16). In the midst of all that is being written and said these days about spirituality and health care, it is surprising that so little has been said about the spiritual lives of physicians and nurses, let alone chaplains. As Heschel reminds us, if health care professionals are to heal patients as whole persons, they themselves must seriously engage the transcendent questions that only persons can ask. If health care professionals are to be true healers, they must rediscover the spiritual meaning of health care.

We have argued that illness is truly a spiritual event. Illness grasps persons by the soul and the body and disturbs them both. Illness raises troubling questions of a transcendent nature—questions about meaning, value, and relationship. How health care professionals answer these questions for themselves will affect the way they help patients struggling with these questions. But patients' suffering and loss will also open health care professionals to their own suffering and loss. In the healing interaction, there is the possibility of transformation of the health care professional and patient by each other. Thus, being present to a patient's suffering can change the clinician—his or her values, priorities, and beliefs can be altered by the experience of another's suffering. In this way the practice of medicine or health care is a dynamic spiritual practice that impacts on the development of the patient and the clinician.

Clinicians today perhaps need to be reminded that if illness is a spiritual event, then the transcendent, healing presence of the divine or sacred can be found right in the midst of the interstices of daily practice—in the infinite space that subsists between their hands and the bodies of the patients they touch. Too few bother to reflect on these matters or talk to each other about them. The transcendent, healing presence of the divine is not only found in explicitly religious conversation with patients who are dying, but in all those countless moments in the office or the hospital in which clinicians communicate meaning and value to their patients and relate to them as persons. Spirituality in practice begins when a clinician becomes aware that illness, injury, and healing operate always on the border between the finite and the infinite—that spiritual place that only persons can apprehend. Ramsey (1970) reminded the world that patients are first and foremost persons. Perhaps it is now time to remind physicians, nurses, and other health care professionals that they are also first and foremost persons.

Barriers to Spirituality in Health Care

Presently multiple barriers stand in the way of the "repersonalization" of health care—this rebirth of health care as a spiritual enterprise. The present economic reconstruction of health care is surely one of these barriers. Reconceptualized to be like any other industry, the chief virtue in health care is no longer compassion, or empathy, or fidelity to trust. The chief virtue of industry is efficiency.

Working in a system in which all parts are considered interchangeable and a patient can see any physician or nurse about any problem in any place at any time, it becomes difficult to believe that questions about relationships have transcendent meaning. In a system in which financial incentives have been reconfigured to make clinicians and patients economic rivals, it is hard for either patients or practitioners to feel that their value constitutes true dignity—that value that has no price, and belongs only to persons (Sulmasy, 2006). In a system in which patient visits have been reduced to seven minutes, it becomes almost unimaginable that questions of meaning can be addressed. Yet these neglected questions of meaning constitute the spiritual in health care.

The spirituality of medical practice must therefore begin with a frank acknowledgment of how much health care professionals are suffering today. Many doctors, nurses, and other health care professionals long to be able to give the spiritual questions of practice the time they deserve. But too many find their efforts thwarted by demands to shorten the time spent with patients, fill out more forms, refer patients to specialists they have never met, and treat them with formulary-approved drugs they have never used.

Nonetheless, clinicians must also be honest about their own part in the current state of affairs. It is true that the industrialization of health care now threatens the spiritual aspects of medical practice from without, denying the importance of the spiritual. Scientific reductionism by health care professionals, however, has equally threatened the spiritual aspects of medical practice from within, by denying the existence of the transcendent.

The fundamental meaning and value of health care, however, can never be altered by science, politics, or economics. The ineradicably interpersonal nature of the healing relationship always begins when one person feels ill, and another, highly skilled and socially authorized, asks, "How can I help you?" Health care is always deeply personal.

It is not easy to be a health care professional today. But when all is said and done, clinicians know that they still touch patients in remarkable ways. The spiritual meaning of health care will outlast all mergers, all managed care organizations, all Medicare and Medicaid cutbacks, all bogus accusations of fraud and abuse, all malpractice suits, all direct-to-consumer advertising, and all manner of profiteering at the expense of patients. If spirituality is real, it is real for times of trial as well as times of triumph. Money can't buy spirituality. And money can't make it go away. In order to provide holistic compassionate care, spirituality must be recognized as an essential element of care in the face of the business of health care.

Each year health care professionals attend the GWish annual renewal retreat in Assisi, Italy, in order to strengthen their own spirituality and integrate it more into their professional lives. Stories are shared about the stresses of health care and how providers can strengthen their abilities to manage stress and work in imperfect environments, yet honor their call to serve others. In the annual George Washington University GWish Summer Institute, health care professionals learn practical tools for integrating spirituality more effectively and for being attentive to their own spiritual needs and cultivate a spiritual practice as part of their professional development.

Spiritual care involves a transformation in how health and illness are viewed. The paradigm is the biopsychosocial-spiritual model in which all dimensions of the person are recognized as equally important. Thus, reimbursement models and health care financing and structure grow out of that model. But even in the current health care system it is possible to practice from this paradigm. Dr. Samuels, a physician in a busy outpatient clinical setting in a city on the East Coast, saw an average of thirty patients per day. One day he was taking a patient history when the patient, Susan, started crying about a recent loss in her life. Dr. Samuels recalls being angry that the tears were disrupting his schedule. After all, Susan had come in for an "acute" visit for a cough. That should be a simple five- to ten-minute visit. But as he listened to her deep suffering, he felt tears well up in his eyes. Her story touched him deeply and awakened a part of him that had been shut down for years. When he asked her what helped her cope in the past, Susan told him about her deep connection to a higher force within the world, a force of goodness and hope. As she spoke, her pain eased and Dr. Samuels' call to help others and bring hope to their lives was reignited. For the first time in many years, he found profound meaning in service to others and remembered the reason he became a doctor and a healer. He recognized that healing included more than technical quick fixes. Healing grows out of the clinical encounter between the patients and the clinician who expresses loving care, support, and commitment to listen to all the patients' concerns, fears, and beliefs. The healing extends beyond the patient. Dr. Samuels was transformed by that encounter and healed in his ability to find new meaning and joy in his work. Dr. Samuels also recognized that spiritual care was not time dependent but rather intention dependent. By shifting his intent to service to the whole person—body, mind, and spirit—his whole encounter became based in compassion. He found he was more effective in establishing rapport, building trust, getting the appropriate diagnosis and treatment plan, and providing better care in the same amount of time. His patients were more satisfied and he was more fulfilled.

Cultivating a Spiritual Practice

How might clinicians cultivate their own spiritual sensibilities? Is it possible to do so in a manner that will be credible in the twenty-first century? Among other ways, we offer the following suggestions. First, if a clinician belongs to a faith tradition, he or she could begin to deepen his or her own spiritual life within that religion. Religion, for some people, makes it easier to grapple with spiritual questions, providing a community of faith and support and a ready-made language with which to describe spiritual struggles and joys. Religion can give a health care professional practices and texts that can be starting points for a deeper exploration of the spiritual life. But spiritual practices may also come from other nonreligious venues such as reading, reflection, yoga, poetry, or art.

Patients struggle with all the big questions. What is the meaning of my illness? Why must I suffer and be punished? Is there anything about me that is valuable now that I am no longer "productive"? What is broken in my relationships that I somehow feel called to fix now that my body is broken? Can my doctor possibly understand what I am really going through? A doctor, nurse, or other health care professional who has begun to explore these questions in his or her own life will be better prepared to help patients struggle with these questions. The world's great religions do not provide simple answers to these questions that are so fundamental to the human condition. Health care professionals who have taken these questions seriously will not trivialize or dismiss the questions of their patients or dispense spiritual bromides to those who struggle with the mysteries of being human in the face of illness and death.

For health care professionals to have authenticity and integrity at the bedside, they must ask themselves the same questions patients and families are asking and grappling with (Kaeton, 1998). Lunn (2004) defines spiritual care in terms of "meeting people where they are and assisting them in connecting or reconnecting to things, practices, ideas, and principles that are at the core of their being—the breath of their life, making a connection between yourself and that person" (p. 154). How can the health care professional meet a patient where he or she is if that caregiver has not explored his or her own life, spirituality, practices, ideas, and principles?

Second, clinicians can cultivate individual spiritual practices. Some clinicians consciously take a few moments in silence before seeing each patient (even between rooms in the outpatient setting) just to become centered and to remind themselves of the sacredness of what they are about to do. Others prayerfully bring their patients to mind at the end of the day. Still others keep spiritual journals of their practices. Some are intentional about appreciating beauty in their lives or taking time in nature to ground themselves. Others have sought out like-minded clinicians and founded group practices that include a period of prayer during the office day. The exact method depends upon the practitioner's personality, spirituality, and circumstances. But some such practice is necessary if one wishes to cultivate one's spiritual life as a practitioner.

Third, clinicians can find fellow health care professionals with whom to engage these questions about spirituality in health care. Some have formed discussion groups in which they read a text about a spiritual topic related to health care and discuss it together—once a month or even more frequently. Some of these groups are interdisciplinary; others are profession-specific. Some even include students.

The spiritual questions are not just for patients. Patients' spiritual or existential struggles can affect the clinicians' journey as well, thus opening the possibility of bidirectional transformation of both parties. Clinicians need to ask themselves, What is the meaning of health care? What is its value? What are right and good healing relationships about? These are spiritual questions that arise for believers and those who do not have specific religious beliefs—for all health care professionals who take both being practitioners and being persons very seriously. Clinicians should also see that asking for spiritual guidance from a chaplain or other spiritual care professional is not a sign of weakness.

We can learn from our patients, but we can also learn from each other. How do we deal with our fallibility? With the deaths of our patients? Can we move beyond complaining about the pressures we now face? Can we see our work as service? Do we ever pray for our patients? Or pray for ourselves as healers? Have we ever experienced the transcendent in our work? Can such peak experiences sustain us?

The transcendent, healing presence of the divine, sacred, or significant can be found in the midst of the interstices of daily practice. It is the time when we begin to recognize that physicians, nurses, and other health care professionals are also first and foremost persons. Without talking about these issues, clinicians might begin to doubt the fundamental soundness of their own spiritual struggles. But if Heschel (Sulmasy, 2006) is right—if to heal a person, one must first be a person—then clinicians must discover what it means for health care itself to be a spiritual practice.

Practice Principles

In the last fifty years there has been some focus on the spiritual caregiver's self-exploration and awareness of his or her strengths and weaknesses so as to be available to enter into a healing relationship with patients and families (Fitchett, 2002). Neil McKenna, chaplain at the Cape Breton Regional Hospital in Sydney, Canada, asserts, "We cannot do for others what we cannot do for ourselves." McKenna suggests that nurses examine six areas of spirituality:

- ► What gives meaning in my life?
- ► What beliefs and values are most important in guiding my life?
- ► What does religion mean to me?
- ► What does spirituality mean to me?
- ► How would a serious, life-threatening illness change the way I find meaning, values, or beliefs in life?

- What spiritual resources do I bring to my work as a nurse or counselor? (e.g., what connection have I made between spirituality and my life experiences of suffering, grief, losses, and such?). (Bryson, 2004)

The National Consensus Project (NCP) Guidelines (2009) state: "Palliative healthcare professionals acknowledge their own spirituality as part of their professional call. They have opportunities to reflect on their beliefs and values as they work with seriously ill and dying patients" (p. 46).

Altruism and Compassion: To Others and to Self

When clinicians respond with altruistic compassion to seriously ill patients, they experience emotions of their own that may overwhelm and deplete their ability to provide quality medical care. Meier et al. (2001) described the emotions of physicians as "to rescue the patient, a sense of failure and frustration when the patient's illness progresses, feelings of powerlessness against illness and its associated losses, grief, fear of becoming ill oneself, or desire to separate from and avoid patients to escape these feelings" (p. 3007). This reaction can not only affect the quality of patient care, but also lead to physician disengagement, burn-out, and diminished ability to provide good care. Many physicians are not trained to identify these emotions or know how to deal with them. The range of emotions for physicians includes professional loneliness, loss of professional sense of meaning and mission, lack of clarity about the scope of medicine, anger at the health care system and medicine in general, loss of the sense of the patient as a human being, and increased risk of burn-out and depression (Meier et al., 2001).

In describing the emotional toll on physicians who care for a patients with cancer, Penson et al. (2000) indicated the strain may lead to feelings of failure and a desire to distance themselves from patients. This may arise from a need to protect themselves from personal harm, and in turn may affect the well-being of both, for example, the patient by virtue of reduced quality of care and the physician by feeling overwhelmed (Figley, 1995). "Compassion fatigue" is a term used to describe the physical, emotional, and spiritual exhaustion of caregiving. Compassion fatigue describes health care professionals becoming exhausted and overwhelmed by their work and then becoming less compassionate to protect themselves (Bryant, 2005).

Compassion fatigue is different than burn-out. Compassion fatigue may lead to burn-out—the development of negative professional attitudes and behaviors as a result of job strain. Work environments can cause job strain when the worker experiences frustration, powerlessness, and an inability to achieve work goals. Burn-out is differentiated from compassion fatigue, as it is a response to the work environment and not to the consequences of caring for people who are suffering. Thus, a health care provider experiencing burn-out has a higher risk for developing compassion fatigue and conversely compassion fatigue can lead to burn-out (Sabo, 2006).

Compassion fatigue may result from the lack of adequate skills in the practice of compassion. Physicians and other health care professionals may in fact be caring, altruistic, and empathic, but they may not practice a compassion that can be sustainable in highly stressful environments with extraordinary or highly intense (frequent) suffering individuals, such as hospice, critical, or long-term care. Clinicians can be empathic, using their intellect to understand what the patient may be experiencing. They may be caring and polite with patients. But compassion calls clinicians into a full experience of the suffering of another without taking on the suffering of another (Puchalski & Lunsford, 2008). Health care professionals must have that ability to be fully present to another person's suffering, but not be overwhelmed or absorbed by the suffering. While health care professionals must be able to take on and share the burdens of others, they must be able to maintain a sense of self that is able to continue to feel hope and joy in each encounter. This entails the ability to continue to focus on the suffering person's feelings and responses, not the health care professional's identification of the suffering as likened to his or her own situation or feelings of isolation or of being the "only one." This is where spirituality becomes so critical. It is the recognition of compassion as a spiritual experience rather than strictly an emotional connection to another. Altruism as agape love is a spiritual love, not dependent on acceptance or recognition from the other. Compassion similarly transcends emotional relationship—it is an altruistic love. The true practice of compassion does not lead to fatigue, as that compassionate practice is grounded in a spiritual practice. In this way the term "compassion fatigue" may be a misnomer. If compassion is practiced fully, and the health care professional has a spiritual practice to support that, there will be no fatigue, as the clinician is trained in a practice of compassion that includes healthy boundaries and self-care.

Meier et al. (2001) propose training for physicians in conscious recognition of their emotions in light of their sense of professional obligation to care for the sick. This training includes being able to recognize and name their feelings or a practice of self-awareness. Then the physician is encouraged to accept the feeling as normal, while reflecting on the emotion and its possible consequences. Finally, the ability to discuss the feelings with trusted colleagues, such as in a hospice team or with other colleagues, enables physicians to confront the emotions, reduce the sense of isolation and despair, and be better able to provide high-quality medical care. Meier et al. (2001), Penson et al. (2000), and others propose that to mitigate the sense of loss and energy depletion by clinicians, it is important that they work within a functional team approach and utilize communication skills, coping methods, and personal reflection strategies to enhance well-being. In addition to self-awareness, clinicians need to have skills in being attentive, that is, being able to focus on the patient and allow distracting thoughts and emotions to be disregarded. Mindfulness is one approach to training in attention, but there are other approaches as well (Puchalski & Lundsford, 2008).

The reality of this threat to the integrity of health care professionals has prompted a new provision in the ANA (2001) Code of Ethics for Nurses: "The nurse owes the same self-regarding duties to self as to others, including the responsibility to preserve integrity and safety, to maintain competence, and to continue personal and professional growth." The threats to integrity of special concern for this provision include the sense that their beliefs and values are not consistent with their behavior, which can undermine their confidence in working with patients and coworkers. It may also alter their ability to communicate and respond compassionately to others. Nurses (and other health care professionals) judge themselves harshly if the outcomes they pursue do not occur, if they are treated with disrespect or punished by other health care professionals or the institution where they practice, or if they fail to act because they lack skills or courage. Interpretive comments regarding this provision for nurses state that "the assault upon their basic values—their understanding of life, death, disability and relationships—may compromise how they perceive the meaning of their work."

When health care professionals are able to respond to their own sense of altruism in their professional work and act out of their own spiritual values and beliefs, it can transform their relationships with patients. In a study of 1,413 family practice patients, McCord et al. (2004) found that 83 percent of patients wanted their physician to ask about their spiritual beliefs. When the physician addresses spirituality, the patient perceives the physician as more compassionate, likely because talking about spiritual issues reflects an interest in the humanity of that patient, relating to the sacred in the other person.

In a study of primary care physician residents, depression was found to be highly prevalent. Those residents who scored higher on a spiritual index and on religious coping were found to have lower rates of depression (Yi et al., 2007). In a GWish program called INSPIR, hospitals are developing initiatives to integrate spirituality more fully into their clinical settings. In addition to tools to help clinicians integrate the implementation model described in this book, health care professionals develop programs to attend to their own spiritual needs, manage their stress in more effective ways, and learn how to practice compassionate presence. In the evaluation of the INSPIR programs, health care professionals who were able to express compassion and attend to their own spiritual needs were also less likely to be burned out (Puchalski & McSkimming, 2006). Thus, by being attentive to one's own spirituality and especially one's sense of sacred call to service to others, clinicians may be able to find more meaning in their work and hence cope better with the stresses of work, as in the case of Dr. Samuels. Once Dr. Samuels reconnected to his greater call—one of service—he began to see his work as a spiritual practice. It enabled him to explore spiritual issues not only with his patients but also with himself. He formed ways to support his work with seriously ill patients by recognizing his ability to make a difference in people's lives. Dr. Samuels developed a gratitude practice. Instead of complaining about the workload and how his patients detracted from his life, he started seeing the richness of his life because of his patients and the relationships he formed with them. His patients were gifts in his life, gifts he treasured and cherished daily.

Recommendations

1. Health care settings should support and encourage the health care professional's attention to self-care, reflection, retreat, and attention to stress management.
    a. The role of spirituality in the health care professional's health, well-being, and resiliency to stress, as well as his or her ability to be compassionate, should be included in training and orientation for new staff members.
    b. Reflective processes should be integrated into regular staff meetings and educational programs using rituals and care resources used for patients.
    c. Environmental aesthetics should encourage reflection and foster self-nurturing behaviors.
2. Professional development should address spiritual development especially as it relates to the health care professional's sense of calling to the profession, the basis of relationship-centered care, and provision of compassionate care.
    a. Provide staff with the resources for basic spiritual care and for addressing spiritual and cultural issues of patients, recognizing how the clinician's own spiritual and cultural background may influence how he or she provides care.
    b. Integrate spirituality and self-care concepts into each profession's curriculum and continuing education programs.
    c. Provide opportunities and resources for health care professionals in their lifelong professional and spiritual growth within the clinical context, recognizing that intimate professional relationships can be transformational for health care professionals and patients.
3. The interprofessional team should be encouraged and given time for regular and ongoing self-examination (e.g., providing a safe, confidential space for compassionate listening at the work site; offering opportunities for off-site retreats; providing resources for referrals [spiritual directors, therapists] as needed).

4. Health care settings should provide opportunities to develop and sustain healthy teams and a sense of connectedness and community. Opportunities may include:
   a. Structured interprofessional teams that honor the voice of all members and value a sense of mutual support.
   b. Ritual and reflections in team meetings.
   c. Provision of on-site staff support for team building.
5. Institutions should provide opportunities for the interprofessional team to discuss ethical issues as they arise:
   a. Health care professionals must be reminded and cautioned regarding the power imbalances that characterize the health care environment. Spirituality should be defined broadly to be inclusive of religious, philosophical, existential, or personal beliefs, values, and practices and centered on patient preferences.
   b. Discussions should include a virtues-based ethics approach to address complex spiritual concerns.
   c. Health care professionals should be afforded the opportunity to discuss spiritual and ethical conflicts and issues they encounter in working with patients and other health care professionals.

12 Quality Improvement

The field of quality improvement (QI) is widely recognized in all settings of health care. The previous decades have witnessed an increased emphasis on improving the quality or performance of health care services through application of standard approaches adapted from business and industry. Well-established QI efforts in health care have addressed common and costly patient care concerns such as patient safety, infection control, relief of common symptoms, patient adherence, and numerous other aspects of patient care delivery. While approaches to QI vary, common features include assessment of the current status of care, planning of strategies for improved care, implementation of strategies, and ongoing evaluation of outcomes with continued refinement of care (Kelly, 2007).

As hospice and palliative care have emerged as major aspects of health care delivery, these settings have adapted QI methods from acute care settings. Hospices have been increasingly pressured to demonstrate effectiveness, and pioneering hospital-based palliative care programs have applied QI strategies to design, implement, and evaluate their services. Common aspects of hospice and palliative care targeted for improvement include relief of pain and symptoms, delivery of bereavement services, patient and family satisfaction with care, use of advanced directives/avoidance of life-prolonging therapies, and ability of these programs to achieve patient goals of care, including achievement of desired place of death (Brunnhuber et al., 2008; Twaddle et al., 2007).

Application of Quality Improvement to Spiritual Care

The spiritual care domain has received less attention than other aspects of palliative care within QI efforts. A goal of this book as the outgrowth of a consensus process is to advance the quality of spiritual care as a critical aspect of palliative care. One way to validate that spiritual care is integral to palliative care is through QI efforts.

There are, however, many challenges to the application of QI efforts in spiritual care. Without well-defined guidelines for spiritual care such as those advanced by NCP, NQF, and this book, it is difficult to have an established standard of quality targeted for improvement. It is also important to acknowledge that the existential quality of spiritual care makes quantification of outcomes a challenge—accessing the relief of suffering, forgiveness, life renewal, meaning in life, and other abstract aspects of spiritual care require approaches far beyond usual quantitative metrics applied to other aspects of palliative care.

Metrics and Methods

Improving the quality of spiritual care and the associated process of QI will require attention to the unique aspects of this domain of care. Some quantitative approaches may be applicable. For example, hospice and palliative care programs can adapt quantitative methods used for areas such as pain to quantify issues such as referrals to chaplaincy, the completion of routine spiritual assessment in the plan of care, and the incorporation of desired rituals into the plan of care or at the time of death.

Qualitative approaches will be needed to capture unique aspects of spiritual care. Data derived from patient, family interviews, staff focus groups, and reflections of patient care will also inform palliative care programs in their quest to improve the quality of spiritual care.

Quality Improvement Frameworks

The NCP Guidelines (2009), NQF Preferred Practices (2006), and recommendations in this book provide a shared framework for palliative care programs and care in general as palliative care is defined as starting from the time someone is diagnosed with a serious illness. There is tremendous opportunity for the spiritual care community to advance this critical aspect of palliative care and medical care in general. Application of these guidelines with vigorous evaluation can advance the field and improve the quality of care received by patients and families. Attention to spiritual care by the NCP and the NQF and other accredited bodies, such as The Joint Commission, can serve to advance spiritual care, without which quality palliative and medical care will not be possible.

Recommendations

1. All palliative care programs should include the domain of spiritual care within their overall quality imporovement plans. Spirituality should be a component of electronic medical records. Clinical settings should monitor the quality of care specifically with regards to spiritual care at the time of death. Measurable outcomes can include patient and staff satisfaction and quality of life. Process measures can include rates of chaplain referral and timelines of completion of routine spiritual assessment among other metrics.

2. Assessment tools should be evaluated to determine which are most efficacious and clinically relevant. Tools and measurement techniques across palliative care settings should be standardized.

3. Quality improvement frameworks based on NCP guidelines that relate to structure, process, and outcomes of spiritual care need to be developed.

4. Building on tested quality improvement models (e.g., pain management), quality imporovement efforts specific to spiritual care should be tested and applied.

5. Research that will contribute to improving spiritual care outcomes to palliative care patients should be supported. Recognizing the complex definition of spirituality and its difficulty in measurement, studies should use multiple quantitative and qualitative methods for evaluation.

6. Funding to evaluate the current state of the science, establish a research agenda, and facilitate research opportunities for spiritual care research should be sought.

13 Conclusion

Spiritual care is an essential domain of quality palliative care as determined by NCP and NQF. Studies have indicated the strong desire of patients with serious illness and end-of-life concerns to have spirituality included in their care. There is a strong empirical and scholarly body of literature to support the inclusion of interprofessional spiritual care as part of a biopsychosocial-spiritual approach to care. Based on the position that palliative care encompasses the care of all patients from the time of diagnosis of serious illness, the principles in this book can be applied to the care of most patients. In this book, practical recommendations are provided for the implementation of interprofessional spiritual care in palliative, hospice, hospital, long-term, and other clinical settings. Critical to the implementation of these recommendations will be interprofessional care that includes board-certified chaplains on the care team, regular ongoing assessment of patients' spiritual issues, integration of patient spirituality into the treatment plan with appropriate follow-up and with ongoing quality improvement, professional education and development of programs, and adoption of these recommendations into clinical site policies.

By utilizing the recommendations set forth in this book, clinical sites can integrate spiritual care models into their programs, develop interprofessional training programs, engage community clergy and spiritual leaders in the care of patients and families, promote professional development that incorporates a biopsychosocial-spiritual practice model, and develop accountability measures to ensure that interprofessional spiritual care is fully integrated into the care of patients.

Some of the future initiatives that will be an outgrowth of this project and are currently being developed by the George Washington Institute for Spirituality and Health, City of Hope, and other organizations are an increased number of training and education programs for health care professionals in interprofessional spiritual care; a "train the trainer" program in spiritual care; more formal opportunities for retreats and reflective programs for clinicians; demonstration projects at hospitals, hospices, and long-term care sites to implement some of the recommendations in this book; and development of spiritual care quality measures. Given the national and international recognition of the importance of spiritual care in clinical care, we hope that clinicians, researchers, and educators will be inspired and affirmed to develop programs that will support spirituality as an essential element of patient-centered, compassionate care.

Acknowledgments

This book brings together the thoughts and contributions of many individuals. Thanks to all the health care professionals who gave their support, shared their wealth of experience, and provided critical review throughout the entire project. The authors also acknowledge the Project Team:

City of Hope, Duarte, CA

Betty R. Ferrell, PhD, MA, FAAN, FPCN; Principal Investigator, Research Scientist

Shirley Otis-Green, MSW, LCSW, ACSW, OSW-C; Senior Research Specialist

Rev. Pam Baird, Spiritual Care Consultant

Rev. Cassie McCarty, MDiv, BCC; Spiritual Care Consultant

Andrea Garcia, BA; Project Coordinator

Rose Virani, RNC, MHA, FPCN, OCN®; Project Director, Senior Research Specialist

George Washington Institute for Spirituality and Health, Washington, DC

Christina Puchalski, MD, MS, FACP, OCDS; Co-Principal Investigator, Executive Director of GWish, Professor of Medicine and Health Sciences, The George Washington University School of Medicine and Health Sciences

Mikhail Kogan, MD; Editor, The Spirituality and Health Online Education and Resource Center (SOERCE); Assistant Professor of Medicine, The George Washington University School of Medicine and Health Sciences

Laurie Lyons, MA; Instructional Designer, The Spirituality and Health Online Education and Resource Center (SOERCE), The George Washington University School of Medicine and Health Sciences

Janet Bull, MA, Associate Director

Laura Kate Zaichkin, Executive Associate

Advisors

Harvey Chochinov, MD, PhD, FRCPC; Professor of Psychiatry; Cancer Care MB; Winnipeg, MB, Canada

George Handzo, MDiv, BCC, MA; Vice President, Pastoral Care Leadership and Practice; The HealthCare Chaplaincy, Inc.; New York, NY

Karen Pugliese, OMA, BCC; Chaplain; Central DuPage Hospital, Winfield, IL

Holly Nelson-Becker, MSW, PhD; Associate Professor, University of Kansas, Lawrence, KS

Maryjo Prince-Paul, PhD, APRN,AHPCN; Assistant Professor, Frances Payne Bolton School of Nursing, Cleveland, OH

Daniel Sulmasy, OFM, MD, PhD; Professor of Medicine and Medical Ethics, School of Medicine and Divinity, University of Chicago, Chicago, IL

Facilitator

M. Brownell "Brownie" Anderson, MEd; Senior Director, Educational Affairs, Association of American Medical Colleges, Washington, DC

Funders

The Project Team is deeply grateful for the Archstone Foundation, Long Beach, California, for their financial support that made this project possible, and members of the Archstone Foundation for their advisory support:

Joseph F. Prevratil, JD; President & CEO

Mary Ellen Kullman, MPH; Vice President

E. Thomas Brewer, MSW, MPH, MBA; Director of Programs

Elyse Salend, MSW; Program Officer

Laura Giles, MSG; Program Officer

Tanisha Metoyer, MAG; Program Associate

Participants

Sandra Alvarez, MD, FAAFP; Family Physician, Elder Health Care of Volusia, Orange City, FL

Lodovico Balducci, MD; Program Leader, Senior Adult Oncology Program, H. Lee Moffitt Cancer Center and Research Institute, Tampa, FL

Tami Borneman, RN, MSN, CNS, FPCN; Senior Research Specialist, City of Hope, Duarte, CA

William Breitbart, MD; Professor and Chief of Psychiatry Service, Memorial Sloan-Kettering Cancer Center, New York, NY

Katherine Brown-Saltzman, RN, MA; Co-Director Ethics Center, The UCLA Health System Ethics Center, Los Angeles, CA

Jacqueline Rene Cameron, MDiv, MD, Episcopal Priest and Attending Physician, St. Joseph's Hospital, Chicago, IL

Ed Canda, MA, MSW, PhD; Director-Research on Spiritual Diversity in S.W., University of Kansas, Lawrence, KS

Carlyle Coash, MA, BCC; Chaplain and NCHPP Section Leader for Spiritual Care, Zen Hospice Project, San Francisco, CA

Rev. Kenneth J. Doka, PhD; Professor, Graduate Gerontology Program, The College of New Rochelle, New Rochelle, NY

Rabbi Elliot Dorff, PhD; Professor in Philosophy, American Jewish University, Los Angeles, CA

James Duffy, MD; Professor of Psychiatry, University of Texas MD Anderson Cancer Center, Houston, TX

Liz Budd Ellmann, MDiv; Executive Director, Spiritual Directors International, Bellevue, WA

George Fitchett, DMin, PhD; Associate Professor and Director of Research, Rush University Medical Center, Chicago, IL

Gregory Fricchione, MD; Associate Chief of Psychiatry, Director, Massachusetts General Hospital, Boston, MA

Roshi Joan Halifax, PhD ; Buddhist Teacher, Zen Priest, and Anthropologist, Upaya Zen Center, Santa Fe, NM

Carolyn Jacobs, MSW, PhD; Dean and Elizabeth Marting Treuhaft Professor, Smith College School of Social Work, North Hampton, MA

Misha Kogan, MD; Assistant Professor of Geriatrics and Palliative Care, George Washington University, Washington, DC

Betty Kramer, PhD, MSW; Professor, School of Social Work, University of Wisconsin—Madison, Madison, WI

Mary Jo Kreitzer, PhD, RN, FAAN; Director, Center for Spirituality and Healing, and Professor, University of Minnesota School of Nursing, Minneapolis, MN

Diane Kreslins, BCC; Spiritual Care Coordinator, Lacks Cancer Center at Saint Mary's Health Care, Grand Rapids, MI

Judy Lentz, RN, MSN, NHA; Chief Executive Officer, Hospice and Palliative Nursing Association, Pittsburgh, PA

Ellen G. Levine, PhD, MPH; Senior Scientist, San Francisco State University, San Francisco, CA

Francis Lu, MD; Professor of Clinical Psychiatry, UCSF, Department of Psychiatry, San Francisco, CA

Brother Felipe Martinez, BA, MDiv, BCC; Roman Catholic Chaplain, Good Samaritan Hospital, Los Angeles, CA

Kristen L. Mauk, PhD, RN, CRRN-A, GCNS-BC; Chair for the Advancement of Nursing Science, Valparaiso University, Valparaiso, IN

Rev. Cecil "Chip" Murray; Retired Pastor, Senior Fellow, Center for Religion, USC, Los Angeles, CA

Rev. Dr. James Nelson, PhD; Senior Minister, Neighborhood Unitarian Universalist Church, Pasadena, CA

Rev. Sarah W. Nichols; Director of Pastoral Care, The Episcopal Home Communities, Alhambra, CA

Steven Pantilat, MD; Professor of Clinical Medicine, UCSF, San Francisco, CA

Tina Picchi, MA, BCC; Director, Palliative Care Services, St. John's Regional Medical Center, Oxnard, CA

Michael Rabow, MD, FAAHPM; Associate Professor of Clinical Medicine, UCSF/Mount Zion, San Francisco, CA

Daniel Robitshek, MD; Professor of Medicine, UC Irvine School of Medicine, Orange, CA

Kay Sandor, PhD, RN, LPC, AHN-BC; Associate Professor, University of Texas Medical Branch, Galveston, TX

Rev. William E. Scrivener, BCC; Senior Director, Department of Pastoral Care, Children's Hospital Medical Center, Cincinnati, OH

Karen Skalla, MSW, ARNP, AOCN; Oncology Nurse Practitioner, Dartmouth Hitchcock Medical Center, Lebanon, NH

Sharon Stanton, MS, BSN, RN; President, Health Ministries Association, Inc., Queen Creek, AZ

Alessandra Strada, PhD; Attending Psychologist, Beth Israel Medical Center, New York, NY

Jeanne Twohig, MPA; Deputy Director, Duke Institute on Care at the End of Life, Durham, NC

External Reviewers

Diane Barrows, OTR, MPA, LCCE; Director, Mission Services, St. Joseph Hospital, Orange, CA

Nancy Berlinger, PhD, MDiv; Deputy Director and Research Scholar, The Hastings Center, Garrison, NY

John Coates, MSW, PhD; Professor, St. Thomas University, Fredericton, NB, Canada

Susan O. Cohen, MA; Pediatric Advanced Illness Care Coordinator, Hackensack University Medical Center, Hackensack, NJ

Eve Cruz, RN, MSN, CNS; Nurse Manager, USC Medical Center, Los Angeles, CA

Farr Curlin, MD; Assistant Professor of Medicine, University of Chicago, Chicago, IL

Eileen Devi Tide; Vice President and Executive Director, Sufi Healing Order, New Lebanon, NY

Ann Marie Dose, PhD, RN, ACNS-BC; Clinical Nurse Researcher, Mayo Clinic, Rochester, MN

Karen Dufault, SP, PhD, MSN, RN; Executive Director, Supportive Care Coalition, Portland, OR

Eileen Dunn, BS; Founder, Warmly Eileen, Wheaton, IL

Linda Dunn, DSN, RN, CNL; Professor of Nursing, University of Alabama, Tuscaloosa, AL

Kathleen Egan-City, MA, BSN; Executive Director, Suncoast Institute, Clearwater, FL

Tim Ford, MA, MS, CT; Palliative Care Chaplain, VCU Massey Cancer Center, Richmond, VA

Auguste H. Fortin VI, MD, MPH, FACP, FAACH; Yale University School of Medicine, New Haven, CT

Sarah Fredricksen, MA, BCC; Hospice Chaplain, Ramona VNA and Hospice, Hemet, CA

Paul Galchutt, BCC, MDiv, Ordained ELCA; Staff and Palliative Chaplain, University of Minnesota Medical Center, Minneapolis, MN

William Gaventa, MDiv; Associate Professor and Director, The Boggs Center, New Brunswick, NJ

Rachel H. Girard, MS, MTS, RN, CDE; Diabetes Nurse Specialist, Maine Medical Center, Portland, ME

Darci L. Graves, MA, PhD; Senior Education Healthcare Specialist , SRA International, Inc., Silver Spring, MD

Marita Grudzen, MHS; Deputy Director, Stanford Geriatric Education Center, Stanford, CA

Tim Hamilton, MDiv; Inpatient Palliative Care Team Chaplain, Kaiser Permanente Los Angeles Medical Center, Los Angeles, CA

Patrick Hansen, MA, BCC; Supervisor Chaplain Services, Mayo Clinic, Phoenix, AZ

Marybeth Harmon, MA, BCC; Director of Spiritual Care, Caritas Norwood Hospital, Franklin, MA

Martha Highfield, PhD, RN; Professor of Nursing, Cal State University of Northridge, Northridge, CA

Eric Holstrom, MDiv, DMin, BCC; Palliative Care and Staff Chaplain, Abington Memorial Hospital, Abington, PA

Alexander Hud, MA, MS; Director of Pastoral Care, Fox Chase Cancer Center, Philadelphia, PA

Ellen L. Idler, PhD; Professor, Rutgers University, New Brunswick, NJ

Arthur H. Jones, DMin, BCC; Staff Chaplain, Hospice of Chattanooga, Chattanooga, TN

Nalini Juthani, MD; Retired Professor, Albert Einstein College of Medicine, Scarsdale, NY

Stephen King, PhD; Manager, Pastoral Care, Seattle Cancer Care Alliance, Seattle, WA

Cynthia Knowles, MDiv; Spiritual Care Counselor, Concord Regional Visiting Nurse Association, Concord, NH

Elaine Lehr, BM, MCM, BCC; Chaplain/Director, Capital Hospice, Falls Church, VA

Claire Levesque, MD; Chief of Neurology, Quincy Medical Center, Quincy, MA

Patricia Levy, PhD, LMSW, ACSW; Associate Professor, Fort Hays State University, Hays, KS

Peggy Matteson, PhD, RN, FCN; Chair, Department of Nursing, Salve Regina University, Newport, RI

Debra Mattison, LMSW, ACSW, BCD, OSW-C; LEO Adjunct Lecturer, University of Michigan Health System, Ann Arbor, MI

Margaret E. McCahill, MD; Professor, UCSD School of Medicine, San Diego, CA

Edith M. Meyerson; Chaplain, Hertzberg Palliative Care Institute, New York, NY

Hellena Moon, BA, AM, MDiv; Doctoral Student, Emory University, Atlanta, GA

Teresa I. Morris, RN, CCM; Reiki Master Practitioner/Teacher, Alpharetta, GA

David Musick, PhD; Associate Dean, Brody School of Medicine, Greenville, NC

Frances Norwood, PhD; Director of Research and Evaluation, Inclusion Research Institute, Washington, DC

Joseph F. O'Donnell, MD; Senior Advising Dean and Director, Dartmouth Medical School, Hanover, NH

Karrie A. Oertli, MDiv, BCC, ACPE; Director, INTEGRIS Baptist Medical Center, Oklahoma City, OK

Penny Phillips, MA, MDiv, BCC; Hospice and Palliative Care Chaplain, Palo Alto Veterans Hospital, Palo Alto, CA

Arturo Roizblatt, MD; University of Chile, Las Condes, Santiago, Chile

Robert Rothemich, BA; Chaplain Resident; Marin General Hospital, Greenbrae, CA

Nola Schmidt, PhD, RN, CNE; Associate Professor; Valparaiso University, Valparaiso, IN

Katrina M. Scott, MDiv, BCC; Oncology Chaplain, Massachusetts General Hospital, Boston, MA

Richard Shannonhouse, MDiv, BCC; Director of Pastoral Care, Memorial Hospital, Jacksonville, FL

Richard W. Smith, MDiv, DMin, BCC; Palliative Care Chaplain, St. Rose Dominican Hospital, Las Vegas, NV

P. Ann Solari-Twadell, RN, PhD, MPA,FAAN; Associate Faculty, Director, Loyola University Chicago, Chicago, IL

Liso Starrett, DMin, BCC; Chaplain, Jansen Hospice and Palliative Care, Tuckahoe, NY

Carol Taylor, RN, MSN, PhD; Director, Center for Clinical Bioethics, Georgetown University, Washington, DC

Kevin F. Tripp, M.Div.; Chaplain, Sutter VNA and Hospice, Santa Rosa, CA

Karen Veronica, MA; Executive Director, Hospice of Morrow County, Mount Gilead, OH

Wendy Wainwright; Manager of Psychosocial Services, Victoria Hospice, Victoria, BC, Canada

G. Jay Westbrook, MS, RN, CHPN; Clinical Director, Compassionate Journey, Lake Balboa, CA

Jacques Weston, MDiv; President, J. Weston Ministries, Hot Springs, AZ

Mary Tederous Williams, PhD, RN; Case Manager, Veterans Administration Western, New York, NY

Sue Wintz, MDiv, BCC; Chaplain, St. Joseph's Hospital and Medical Center, Phoenix, AZ

Abebaw Yohannes, PhD, MSc; Reader in Physiotherapy, Manchester Metropolitan University, Manchester, United Kingdom

Michael R. Young, MDiv; Hospice Chaplain, retired, Community Hospice, Catskill, NY

Anne Christine Zook, RN, BSN, MA; Palliative Medicine Coordinator, Mercy Medical Center, Des Moines, Iowa

Appendix A Definitions Related to Spiritual Care

There are many definitions in the literature used for spirituality, religion, spiritual care, and related items. This poses a difficulty when trying to compare findings from research or to establish universally applicable clinical guidelines. Below are key definitions found in the literature.

Spirituality

1. Spirituality refers to the propensity to make meaning through a sense of relatedness to dimensions that transcend the self in such a way that empowers and does not devalue the individual. This relatedness may be experienced interpersonally (as connectedness within oneself), intrapersonally (in the context of others and the natural environment), and transpersonally (referring to a sense of relatedness to the unseen, God, to power greater than self and ordinary sources). (Reed, 1992)

2. Spirituality speaks to what gives ultimate meaning and purpose to one's life. It is that part of people that seeks healing and reconciliation with self or other. (Puchalski, 2006c)

3. Spirituality can be understood in six domains based on the review of the literature:

   ► Essence: The core of one's being, the source of one's humanity, a way of being and experiencing life that comes through a transcendent dimension
   ► Meaning:
      ► Ultimate meaning—that defines in relation to a transcendence, sacred, or divine.
      ► Meaning—in life, gives purpose
   ► Transcendence: An awareness of something greater than oneself; sacred, divine, God, higher power, energy force
      ► Relationship: Connection to self, others, God, sacred, nature
   ► Values: Beliefs, morals, standards that guide one in life; experiential appreciation of beauty, love, nature
   ► Rituals, spiritual practices: External expression of spirituality, method of transformation, expansion of self. (Puchalski, 2006c)

4. Spirituality provides a source of meaning and a way to understand the significance of living. Aspects of spirituality include the need for purpose and meaning, forgiveness, love, relatedness, hope, and creativity and its expression. It may include rituals, music, prayer, and symbolic representations to help understand or interpret what it means to be human and to reckon with things greater than us.

5. Spirituality is recognized as a factor that contributes to health in many persons. The concept of spirituality is found in all cultures and societies. It is expressed in an individual's search for ultimate meaning through participation in religion and/or belief in God, family, naturalism, rationalism, humanism, and the arts. All of these factors can influence how patients and healthcare professionals perceive health and illness and how they interact with one another. (AAMC, 1999)

6. Spirituality is defined in terms of personal views and behaviors that express a sense of relatedness to a transcendent dimension or to something greater than self. (Reed, 1987)

7. Spirituality is a way of being and experiencing that comes about through the awareness of a transcendent dimension. Spirituality is characterized by certain identifiable values in regard to self, others, nature, life and whatever one considers to be the Ultimate. . . . It is that which gives one purpose, meaning, and hope and provides a vital connection. (Elkins et al., 1988)

8. At its most basic level, spirituality can be seen as the very essence of who we all are as human beings. It is that dimension that brings meaning to our lives. (Frankl, 1963)

9. Spirituality: An inner belief system. It is a delicate "spirit-to-spirit" relationship to oneself and others, and the God of one's understanding. (Joint Commission Resources, 2005)

10. Spirituality can be defined as a complex and multidimensional part of the human experience—our inner belief system. It helps individuals to search for the meaning and purpose of life, and it helps them experience hope, love, inner peace, comfort, and support. (Joint Commission, 2005)

11. Spirituality is often a broad concept, referring to the human search for a sense of meaning, purpose, and morality in the context of relationships with self, others, the universe, and ultimate reality. (Joint Commission, 2005)

12. Spirituality is a "sense of inner-connectedness with a feeling of purpose and meaning in life, which enables transcendence over immediate circumstances." (Pargament, 1997)

13. The spiritual typically incorporates the human quest for meaning, purpose, and an ethical ground; it stands in relation to an individual's deepest or most central beliefs and experiences about the nature of reality. (Canda & Smith, 2001).

14. Spiritual awareness develops across time through relationships with one's inner self, others, the universe and ultimate reality, whatever a person understands this to be. It may or may not include religious practice and beliefs. Spirituality may be perceived as the core essence of an individual or it may encompass the other biopsychosocial domains. Fundamentally, the spiritual is an integrative, holistic component of life that may also include experiences of a transpersonal nature. (James, 1905; Tillich, 1963)

Religion

1. The externals of one's belief system: church, prayers, traditions, rites, and rituals, among others. (Joint Commission Resources, 2005)

2. Religion refers to a belief system to which an individual adheres. Religion involves particular rituals and practices—the externals of our belief system. . . . Not everyone is religious, nor is religion a requirement for spirituality. (Joint Commission Resources, 2005)

3. A system of organized beliefs and worship that the person practices. (Emblen, 1992)

4. Religion usually refers to an organized system of spiritual beliefs, behaviors, rituals and ethical principles shared by a community and conveyed over time. (Canda & Furman, 1999)

5. An individual who is religious may or may not see himself/herself as spiritual. Social work also understands that some individuals express an extrinsic form of religion which is related to the primary importance of social engagement and maintaining social relationships expressed through religious affiliation. (Nelson-Becker, 2003)

6. Generally, religion is thought of as the institutions, and participation in those institutions, in which the members have shared ideology of the divine or sacred. (Burke, 2006)

Existential

1. Of or relating to one's existence or purpose. ("Existential," 2009)

2. Going beyond self, the body, and other human beings. It can convey a sense of being part of a greater whole, of communion with a Higher Power or Higher Being. (Prince-Paul, 2008)

3. Existential refers to a philosophical approach where one's primary task is to find what determines one's own level of meaning in life. Often this may involve an anguished process where prior beliefs no longer seem valid and one begins a journey to find one's own meaning in life. Meaning is often conceived in a way that is personal and acknowledges that others may hold other quite different meanings. At the end of life, terminally ill individuals may expand their curiosity in the hope that this will lead to new self-discovery. This often takes an individual through a process of uncertainty and ambiguity that includes the re-examination of prior understandings to determine what one holds for the self to be true. (Nelson-Becker, 2006)

Spiritual Well-Being

1. Occurs through a dynamic and interactive growth process that leads to a realization of the ultimate purpose and meaning of life. (Hungelmann et al., 1996)

2. Ability to experience and integrate meaning and purpose in life through connectedness with self, others, art, music, literature, nature, and/or a power greater than oneself that can be strengthened. (Johnson et al., 2006)

3. Spiritual well-being is the affirmation of life in a relationship with God, self, community and environment that nurtures and celebrates wholeness. (NICA, 1975)

Suffering

1. Suffering is the state of distress brought about by an actual or perceived threat to the integrity or continued existence of the whole person. Suffering is "an anguish that is experienced, not only as a pressure to change, but as a threat to our composure, our integrity, and the fulfillment of our intentions." (Cassell, 1991)

2. Pain + fear = suffering. (Otis-Green, 2007)

Spiritual Care

1. Pastoral Care—spiritual/religious care delivered by a professional chaplain focusing on spiritual/religious needs and resolving spiritual/religious issues that impede coping.

2. Intuitive, interpersonal, altruistic, and integrative expression that is contingent in the nurse's awareness of the transcendent dimension of life but reflects the patient's reality. (Sawatzky & Pesut, 2005)

3. Interventions, individual or communal, that facilitate the ability to express the integration of the body, mind, and spirit to achieve wholeness, health, and a sense of connection to self, others, and a higher power. (ANA & HMA, 2005)

4. Client care that recognizes and supports the holistic need for healing. Spiritual care involves attention to the needs of the soul for compassion (both giving and receiving love), meaning/purpose, hope, faith, and reconciliation. It involves initiating an assessment to determine if spirituality and/or religion are important to a patient and then, if so, including these aspects in treatment in whatever manner is both important to the client and ethical. In social work, we use the term "spiritually-sensitive practice" to include a concern for practitioners to listen to spiritual cues. Many times, the spiritual discourse has been a hidden discourse and while it may be personally important to individuals, the value of it will not be revealed unless a patient is explicitly asked. This has often been the case for members of minority and/or marginalized cultures. (Nelson-Becker, 2003)

Spiritual Values

Meaning is understood as the worth of life. Having a sense of accomplishment—based on having assumed roles such as being a spouse, parent or child, creative activities or vocational roles—is fundamental to a coherent sense of feeling whole. Attention to things unknowable about the cosmos and nature can engender awe and reverence for the sacred. Spirituality will be a powerful source of meaning for many; faith in religious beliefs a consolation for others. (Breitbart et. al., 2008)

Hope is a belief in a positive outcome related to events and circumstances in one's life. Hope is the feeling that what is wanted can be had or that events will turn out for the best. ("Hope," 2009)

Faith is a belief in the trustworthiness of an idea. Formal usage of the word "faith" is usually reserved for concepts of religion, as in theology, where it almost universally refers to a trusting belief in a transcendent reality, or else in a Supreme Being and said being's role in the order of transcendent, spiritual things. ("Faith," 2009)

Purpose: One needs something to believe in, something for which one can have whole-hearted enthusiasm. One needs to feel that one's life has meaning, that one is needed in this world. (Senesh & Piercy, 2004)

Reconciliation: At the most basic level, reconciliation is all about individuals. It cannot be forced on people. They have to decide on their own whether to forgive and reconcile with their one-time adversaries. (Hauss, 2003)

Social connectedness is a psychological term used to describe the quality and number of connections we have with other people in our social circle of family, friends and acquaintances. These connections can be both in real life, as well as online. The more socially connected a person is in their lives, generally the greater sense of self-control and self-determination they feel. ("Social connectedness," 2009)

Dignity is "the quality or state of being worthy, honored, or esteemed." ("Dignity," 2009)

Dignity conveys the notion of the inherent respect due to patients who are preparing for death. (Chochinov et al., 2002)

Spiritual Distress

Spiritual distress refers to the impaired ability to experience and integrate meaning and purpose in life through connectedness with self, others, art, music, literature, nature, and/or a power greater than oneself. (NANDA International, 2007)

Spiritual distress is evidenced by:

- Questioning the credibility of his/her belief system.
- Demonstrating discouragement or despair.
- Unable to practice usual religious rituals.
- Ambivalent feelings (doubts) about beliefs.
- Expressing that he/she has no reason for living.
- Feeling a sense of spiritual emptiness.
- Showing emotional detachment from self and others.
- Expressing concern, anger, resentment, fear—over the meaning of

life, suffering, death.

- ▸ Requesting spiritual assistance for a disturbance in belief system. (RN Central Online, 2007)

Despair: to lose all hope and confidence. ("Despair," 2009)

Guilt/Shame: Guilt says I've done something wrong; shame says there is something wrong with me. Guilt says I've made a mistake; shame says I am a mistake. Guilt says what I did was not good; shame says I am no good. (Bradshaw, 1988)

Meaninglessness was directly related to death: If we all must die, can life have any ultimate meaning? (Park, 2007)

Demoralization is experienced as a persistent inability to cope, together with associated feelings of helplessness, hopelessness, meaninglessness, subjective incompetence and diminished self-esteem. Demoralization syndrome is defined as "a psychiatric state in which hopelessness, helplessness, meaninglessness, and existential distress are the core phenomena." (Kissane et al., 2001)

Isolation: Social withdrawal. (Health Grades, 2009)

Spiritual pain is an individual's perception of hurt or suffering associated with that part of his or her person that seeks to transcend the realm of the material; it is manifested by a deep sense of hurt stemming from feeling of loss or separation from one's God or deity, a sense of personal inadequacy or sinfulness before God and man; or a pervasive condition of loneliness of spirit. (O'Brien, 1999)

Spiritual Community

Group of interacting people who share characteristics with relation to spiritual, cultural, ethnic, or moral values. (McDonald, 2006)

Group of people united by shared spiritual values, who gather together in support of the expression of their spiritual values and practices. (O'Donnell, 2007)

Appendix B   Sample Spiritual Histories and Assessments

FICA   A Spiritual History

F   Faith and Belief

I   Importance

C   Community

A   Address in Care or Action

F   "Do you consider yourself spiritual or religious?"
- or –
"Do you have spiritual beliefs that help you cope with stress (contextualize to the situation, for e.g. with what you are going through right now, with dying, with dealing with pain)?"
If the patient responds "No" the physician might ask, "What gives your life meaning?"

Sometimes patients respond with answers such as family, career, or nature. Patients who respond "yes" to the spiritual question should also be asked about meaning.

I   "What importance does your faith or belief have in your life? Have your beliefs influenced how you take care of yourself in this illness? What role do your beliefs play in regaining your health?" "Do your beliefs influence your decisions about your health care?"

These questions can help lead into questions about advance directives and proxies who can represent the patient's beliefs and values. One can also ask about spiritual practices and rituals that might be important to people, or dietary restrictions based on beliefs.

C   "Are you part of a spiritual or religious community? Is this of support to you and how? Is there a group of people you really love or who are important to you?"

Communities such as churches, temples, and mosques, or a group of like-minded friends can serve as strong support systems for some patients

A   "How would you like me, your health care provider, to address these issues in your health care?" Or ask the patient, "What action steps do you need to take in your spiritual journey?"

Often it is not necessary to ask this question but to think about what spiritual issues need to be addressed in the treatment plan. Examples include referral to chaplains, pastoral counselors, or spiritual directors, journaling, and music or art therapy. Sometimes the plan may be simply to listen and support the person in his or her journey.

(Puchalski & Romer, 2000)

S	Spiritual belief system	Do you have a formal religious affiliation? Can you describe this? Do you have a spiritual life that is important to you? What is your clearest sense of the meaning of your life at this time?
P	Personal spirituality	Describe the beliefs and practices of your religion that you personally accept. Describe those beliefs and practices that you do not accept or follow. In what ways is your spirituality/religion important to you? How is your spirituality/religion important to you in daily life?
I	Integration with a spiritual community	Do you belong to any religious or spiritual groups or communities? How do you participate in this group/community? What is your role? What importance does this group have for you? In what ways is this group a source of support for you? What type of support and help does or could this group provide for you in dealing with health issues?
R	Ritualized practices and restrictions	What specific practices do you carry out as part of your religious and spiritual life (e.g., prayer, meditation, service, etc.)? What lifestyle activities or practices does your religion encourage, discourage, or forbid? What meaning do these practices and restrictions have for you? To what extent have you followed these guidelines?
I	Implications for medical care	Are there specific elements of medical care that your religion discourages or forbids? To what extent have you followed these guidelines? What aspects of your religion/spirituality would you like to keep in mind as we care for you? What knowledge or understanding would strengthen our relationship as physician and patient? Are there barriers to our relationship based upon religious or spiritual issues? Would you like to discuss religious or spiritual implications of health care?
T	Terminal events planning	Are there particular aspects of medical care that you wish to forgo or have withheld because of your religion/spirituality? Are there religious or spiritual practices or rituals that you would like to have available in the hospital or at home? Are there religious or spiritual practices that you wish to plan for at the time of death, or following death? From what source do you draw strength in order to cope with this illness?

(Maugans, 1996)

H	Sources of hope, strength, comfort, meaning, peace, love, and connection
O	The role of organized religion for the patient
P	Personal spirituality and practices
E	Effects on medical care and end-of-life decisions

(Anandarajah & Hight, 2001)

The Spiritual History Scale (SHS-4)

Would you tell me for each of the following statements, whether you strongly agree, somewhat agree, neither agree nor disagree, somewhat disagree, or strongly disagree?

God Helped

God has helped me this far through my life. (GOD_HELP)

Some of the good things that have happened to me were blessings from God. (BLESSING)

When I was about sixty, I looked for God's guidance in my daily life. (GUIDE_60)

Overall, God has answered my prayers. (ANSWER)

I have trusted God to take care of me through the years. (TRUSTGOD)

Through the years I have prayed for my health and for the health of others. (PRAYHLTH)

Overall, my religious life has taught me to have a positive attitude. (POSITIVE)

Overall, my religious life has helped me to reduce stress. (LOWERSTR)

Overall, my religious life has helped me to persevere (go on when life gets hard). (PERSEVER)

I have lived this long because God's time for me to die has not yet come. (LIV_TIME)

Lifetime Religious Social Support

For most of my life, my social life has revolved around the church (synagogue). (SOCIAL_C)

For most of my life, I have known many of the people in my church (synagogue) well. (KNOW WELL)

An important part of my religious life has been inviting and taking people to my church (synagogue). (INVITE)

When I was fifty, I was very involved in the church (synagogue). (INVOLV50)

Family History of Religiousness

When I was a child, I was very involved in the church (synagogue). (INVOLVCH)

When I was a child, the church (synagogue) was like family to me. (FAM_CH)

When I was a child, religion was a natural part of my life. (NATURAL)

When I was a child, my parents left my religion up to me. (LEFT_UP)

When I was a young child, I had a religious or spiritual role model. (ROLE_CH)

My family passed down their religion to me. (FAM_PASS)

Cost of Religiousness

At times, my religious life has caused conflict between myself and other people. (CONFLICT)

At times, my religious life has caused me stress. (CAUSESTR)

I have suffered physically because of my religion (SUFFER)

(Hays et al., 2001)

University of California San Diego Medical Center

PATIENT SPIRITUAL ASSESSMENT FORM

Patient:_____ Date: _____

Phone Assessment ❏   Patient Visit ❏

Spiritual Care Refused: ❏ Yes   ❏ No

Does Patient/Family Request Faith Community Contacted   ❏ Yes   ❏ No

Patient's Religious Identity/History: _____

Pastor ❏   Priest ❏   Rabbi ❏   Other:_____

Name: _____   Phone:_____

Family Member's Name	*Relationship to Patient*
_____	_____
_____	_____
_____	_____
_____	_____

Significant Anniversaries: ❏ Yes   ❏ No   If yes, specify_____

Significant Birthdays: ❏ Yes   ❏ No   If yes, specify_____

Tell about illness and how it has affected your life:_____

_____

_____

What are your worries or concern?_____

_____

_____

What has life been I like for you?_____

_____

_____

What has given you meaning, strength, or enjoyment?

❏ Work   ❏ Role:_____

❏ Family   ❏ Hobbies:_____

❏ Significant Relationships ❏ Music:_____

❏ Prayer   ❏ Nature:_____

❏ Other: _____

SPIRITUAL PAIN ASSESSMENT FORM

PATIENT NAME:_____

ROOM NUMBER:_____

Date:_____

Meaning Pain Scale

1	2	3	4	5
life is filled with w/purpose & meaning	life is good, I know what I want to accomplish	I feel generally motivated	I lack energy to accomplish	life has become meaningless

Comments:_____

Relatedness Pain Scale

1	2	3	4	5
I feel a strong sense of connection w/ the person & things that matter to me	I feel connection with those important to me	Most important areas of my life seem balanced	I feel some disassociation from key relationships/ issues	I feel seriously alienated from someone/ thing that is important to me

Comments:_____

Forgiveness Pain Scale

1	2	3	4	5
I feel a deep sense of reconciliation toward myself and others	I'm unaware of unresolved issues	There are no outstanding issues that are calling for forgiveness in my life	I know of areas I need to work on to forgive others	I feel a strong sense of unforgiving toward myself/ others

Comments:_____

Hope Pain Scale

1	2	3	4	5
I feel hope-filled optimistic	I sense all will probably work out positively	I generally trust what the future holds for me	I sometimes question "why me?"	I am experienc-ing deep depression & hopelessness

COMMENTS:_____

_____

_____

CAREGIVER'S OBSERVATIONS:_____

_____

(Adapted from assessment tool designed by Richard Grove, St. Charles Medical Center, Bend, OR.)

Spiritual Care Assessment

Faith group: _____ Particular affiliation: _____

Pastor:_____ Phone: _____

Patient/family_____ gives consent to contact Pastor: ❏ Yes   ❏ No

Areas to address

1. What is the patient's/family's source of strength?

2. What relationships have been significant in the past and at this time?

3. What group or organization has been important for providing strength?

4. What network will be available at home?

5. What are the spiritual needs at this time and how can the chaplain be of help?

Theological issues

1. Image of God: _____

2. Relationship with God:_____

3. Important spiritual resources: ❏ Prayer   ❏ Scripture   ❏ Sacraments
   ❏ Worship   ❏ Other: _____

Spiritual issues to address (use back of form if necessary):

Proposed spiritual component of Care Plan (use back of form if necessary):

Chaplain's signature_____ Date_____

Fairview Health Services
Spiritual Assessment
Brief Outline

Six Components of a Spiritual Care Assessment for Palliative Care Patients

- What spiritual practices are life-giving for you?
- What gives you hope and meaning?
- Indicate your faith community/spiritual group membership and its significance.
- Who are your spiritual mentors and guides?
- Have you made plans for spiritual care at the end of your life? Have you talked with anyone about those plans?
- Do you have spiritual concerns or issues you need to address? (i.e., confession, forgiveness, reconciliation, anointing, letting go, closure)

Spiritual Assessment: Examples of Questions to Begin Dialogue

1. What gives you hope and meaning?
   - The last time you were very sick, what nurtured and sustained you?
   - To what do you turn to help you through tough times?
     Goal: To identify if spirituality/religion is on the patient's/family radar.
2. If # 1 is a yes, identify the community.
3. Who are the preferred spiritual care providers?
4. What are the spiritual issues the patient/family are addressing?
5. What are the desired outcomes of the spiritual care plan?

Keep documentation as succinct as possible

(Palliative Care, University of Minnesota Medical Center, Fairview)

Appendix C Examples of Spiritual Screening Questions That Can Be Integrated into Hospital Intake Forms

1) Are there cultural or spiritual issues we need to address?
(from Chevy Chase Endoscopy Center)

2) Do you have any spiritual beliefs that would affect your care?
❏ Yes ❏ No
(from Virginia Hospital Center Emergency Department Nursing Record)

3) Cultural/Spiritual Beliefs/Practices that influence treatment, medications, care: ❏ No ❏ Yes (list):_____

4) Religion: Desires to see Clergy: ❏ No ❏ Yes—Referred
(from Cedars-Sinai Medical Center Patient Profile Medical–Surgical)

Spiritual Needs   1) Spiritual Comfort Assessment
Spiritual supports
Spiritual needs and/or distress

2) Spiritual Support: Referral to Chaplain
Provide opportunity for expression of beliefs,
fears, and hopes
Provide access to religious resources
Facilitate religious practices

(Beth Israel Health Care System)

Appendix D Spirituality Cases

Case 1: "My Life Is Meaningless"

Ms. Harper is a seventy-five-year-old former advocate for the home-less, who recently suffered a stroke that left her with mild cognitive impairment and hemiparesis. The meaning in her life came from her work, and since the stroke she is unable to work and feels life has no meaning anymore.

Spiritual History

F	Atheist; meaning in social activism.
I	Work is her life and her whole sense of who she is.
C	Activist community.
A	Interested in passing on her dreams to younger people who will carry on her work when she dies. Referral to pastoral counselor, find resources for patient to work with students, continued presence, journaling (patient may be interested in recording her narrative or history).

Interventions

The goal is to help Ms. Harper move beyond defining herself by what she did to a deeper intrinsic meaning and value of herself as a person. Cognitive-oriented therapy can help. One can ask questions such as:

- What have been important events in your life?
- What is the most important event in your life?
- Have you loved and have you been loved?

For religious patients, one can explore their relationship with God and whether the relationship with God or religious belief provides a sense of peace or meaning in their lives. For nonreligious patients, one can explore whether the spiritual or other belief provides peace, meaning, or hope. By reflective listening, try to guide people to look at all the dimensions of their lives. One can help people see problems in their lives as goals and sources of meaning. Sometimes people find meaning in their struggle, sometimes not. But as caregivers, we can support them in looking beyond the extrinsic and into an intrinsic sense of value in themselves and find some meaning in their struggle.

Finally, one can consider referral to a cognitive therapist, chaplain, pastoral counselor, and spiritual director. For Ms. Harper, she is not interested in these resources but is interested in pursuing teaching of the next generation and any resources and community connections that can help her with that.

Case 2: "Hopelessness"

Ronda is a fifty-eight-year-old female with end-stage ovarian cancer. Seven and a half years after multiple surgeries and chemotherapy with good outcomes, she is now faced with advanced disease for which there is no longer any treatment. Her hope has always been for a cure. Now she faces a deep sense of hopelessness.

Hope can be expressed in many ways. It may initially be for a cure, but when that is no longer possible, people may still find hope in finding important projects, making peace with others, and having a peaceful death.

Spiritual History

F	Raised Jewish culturally; meaning has always been in nature and not in religion.
I	Spirituality is important, and now that she is dying she would like to know how Judaism views dying and what rituals might help her.
C	Friends are her spiritual support.
A	Would like to see a rabbi to discuss her spiritual questions with him. Referral to chaplain to help connect patient with rabbi, dream list, explore sources of hope.

Interventions

- Help patient create a dream list
- Talk about the relationships in the person's life—is there any conflict from relationships?
- What are the person's sources of hope? What have they been in past life experiences in times of stress?
- If person is religious, what does his or her religion say about hope? Is that meaningful to the person?

For this patient, part of the plan would be to refer her to a rabbi, and help with accomplishing dreams as much as possible with referral to appropriate resources.

Case 3: "Despair"

Katie is a forty-six-year-old female with metastatic breast cancer. She is married, with two children, ages thirteen and fifteen. Her goal has been to live to see both children graduate from high school and start college. In the last two months, she has had a rapid decline. When confronted with the possibility of dying, she expresses deep despair about her life. In particular, she feels as if her life is being cut too short and that God may not be there for her. Of greatest concern is what will happen to her children. Her own mother died of breast cancer when she was sixteen; she does not want to cause the same suffering to her children.

Spiritual History

F	Catholic; meaning in family and in God and Mary. Mary is a model for her in being a "Mother who suffered."
I	Very important in her life but feels God has let her down and no longer supports her. She does not want aggressive care at the end of life; does want "last rites."
C	Strong church community but feels awkward about their visits. She feels extreme fatigue.
A	Wants a priest to visit her for "last rites" but feels afraid he will judge her about her questions about God.
	Referral to chaplain who could help coordinate sacraments as well as do spiritual counseling, continued presences, explore sources of hope, family meeting.

Interventions

- ▸ Listening, presence
- ▸ Ask about relationships with family, God, and church members
- ▸ Ask about sources of hope or how spiritual beliefs have helped in times in her life that were difficult and painful
- ▸ Validate her feelings as normal
- ▸ Explore ways of conveying her concerns for her children to her family
- ▸ Explore if community member visits can be helpful in the midst of her fatigue (i.e., not having to entertain visitors, but allowing simply their presence)

The plan here would be referral to a chaplain, priest visit for sacraments, continued presence and support, and recommend family meeting to talk about death and dying issues.

Case 4: Compliance with Treatment

Brenda is a forty-two-year-old female, mother of six children. Her partner of twelve years is arrested for drug possession. While in jail, she finds out he is HIV positive. Brenda comes to a walk-in clinic and asks to be tested. On a follow-up visit, the doctor tells her that she is HIV positive. Brenda responds, "God, why are you doing this to me?" The doctor proceeds by telling her that she is in an early stage of the infection, that there are new medications, and that there is good reason to believe that she can live for many years with this chronic illness. But Brenda proceeds with cries to God, "Why are you punishing me?" She refuses to do more tests and to pursue treatment. The physician obtains a spiritual history:

Spiritual History

F	Nondenominational Christian; her children are what give her life meaning.
I	Very important in her life, prays daily, attends Bible study Wednesday evenings and services on Sunday.
C	Active in her church, worries about going to church as she believes her illness is a punishment from God for having had an abortion at age twelve after a relative raped her.
A	Referral to pastoral counselor, invite Brenda's clergy to next visit to discuss illness and spiritual issues.

Intervention
- ▸ Listening to patient's story without judgment
- ▸ Referral to a pastoral counselor who could explore the emotional issues of being raped as a child, and the spiritual issues that have resulted in Brenda's interpretation of her illness as punishment
- ▸ Offer an invitation to Brenda to bring her minister to the office to discuss some of the medical issues and how her spirituality is affecting her understanding of her illness
- ▸ Consider a forgiveness intervention

It is not uncommon for patients to interpret their illness as a punishment from God, or a curse or bad karma. The clinician may not agree with the interpretation but should respect the patient and the patient's beliefs. For the clinician the task is to not to change the perspective of the patient but to listen to the beliefs and then provide appropriate resources to help the patient gain a deeper understanding of where those beliefs are coming from. This process could result in a reframing for the patient of the situation or a deeper conviction that what he or she believes is correct. In some cases, rituals or forgiveness interventions can be helpful. Forgiveness has been shown to have positive health benefits. Working with spiritual care professionals is critical in these cases.

The plan here would be referral to a pastoral counselor or invite her clergy to the clinical office and continued presence and support.

Case 5: "Why Is This Happening . . . ?"

Michala is a forty-five-year-old artist undergoing chemotherapy for metastatic breast cancer. She has been coping well with her illness but recently developed nausea and vomiting related to her chemotherapy. She became dehydrated and needed to be treated at the emergency department. The following day she goes to her primary care office and sees the nurse practitioner. She says to her, "Why is all of this happening?"

The nurse practitioner asks Michala to tell her more. Michala tells her provider that this particular episode at the emergency department made her realize she will one day die from her cancer.

F	Believes in God or a higher power but is no longer religious; meaning is derived from her art. Her art helps her experience the transcendent.
I	Her painting is the essential element of her life; her paintings are her legacy and she hopes to live long enough to finish an art show in New York. She expresses concern that chemotherapy will interfere with that.
C	Used to be Episcopalian but that is no longer important to her; her spiritual group consists of her colleagues in an art group she belongs to.
A	Work with oncologist to adjust chemotherapy to allow Michala to have the energy and ability to finish her artwork and attend the art show in New York. Invite patient to consider formal ways to make her paintings a legacy. Continued presence; consider a chaplain referral.

Intervention

Meaning can be derived from many sources; art is one way. In this case, the patient's quality of life is closely tied to her ability to paint and exhibit. Adjusting medical treatment to help her accomplish her goals is very important. Legacy building is also an important intervention in end-of-life care.

The plan for this patient would be to work with her medical team to help Michala accomplish her goals. Her clinicians should also continue to provide compassionate presence and to continue to reassess her goals for treatment and her life. A chaplain referral can also be considered.

Case 6: Breaking Bad News

Raymond is a Crohn's disease patient who is coming to the doctor's office to discuss results from a routine screening colonoscopy done one week ago. Biopsies showed dysplasia in the cecum, the transverse colon, and the sigmoid colon. An upper GI X-ray, done two months ago, showed extensive scarring in the ileum. The patient's disease began twenty-five years ago with diarrhea, abdominal cramping, and weight loss. The patient has been treated with Asacol with good response—no major flares for the past three years; has normal bowel movements and no cramping. Patient has had some back and joint pains, which the patient was told might be part of the disease.

The doctor breaks the news to Raymond and recommends a total colectomy. Raymond's normal coping style is one of humor, but upon hearing the bad news, he goes from jocular to stunned: "I've been through so many of these, they've gotten to be so routine—I never thought anything bad would be found. You know, I always told myself I would rather die than live with a bag!"

Spiritual History

F	Buddhist
I	Buddhism is a way of life for him. He finds peace when he is able to view stressful challenges within the Buddhist context—realizing that nothing in life is permanent and that stress comes from becoming overly attached. He sometimes must struggle to apply this framework—his first inclination sometimes is to panic.
C	Attends a Buddhist temple for teachings and meditation practices.
A	He recognizes how he alternates between panic and calming himself and asks the physician to remind him of his spiritual practice when he gets panicked. He also asks if he can go on a five-day Buddhist retreat and then make a decision about his treatment once he returns.

Intervention

Spirituality can impact the way people cope with serious news. In this case, Raymond has panicked at the thought of having a colectomy. But this news also is a setback for him and likely raises issues of grief and fear about the future. He has a spiritual practice that has helped him with difficult times in the past. He recognizes that this coping resource could help him in the current situation to make a decision that he is comfortable with.

The plan would therefore be to acknowledge his beliefs and practices, delay a decision on the surgery, if safe, until after the retreat.

Case 7: Demoralization

Eric Jenkins is a thirty-four-year-old male with a past medical history of depression. He has had some treatment for his depression and is prescribed medications, which he is currently not taking. He presents to the Emergency Department with the complaint of wanting to jump off a highway bridge into traffic and kill himself. "What am I living for?" He says he does not see a reason for taking his medications.

Eric has been the sole caregiver of his elderly mother and father for about ten years. He tells the ER doctor that taking care of his parents has been "his life." His father died about four years ago. He continued taking care of his mother after his father died but was devastated six months ago when his mother died. He says that now "I have no purpose to my life." He did not leave a suicide note.

He looks very sad and continues to gaze downward. When he does look at you, his eyes clearly show that he is asking for help. The doctor does a full assessment and does not find Eric to be at risk for suicide. He has minimal vegetative signs of depression.

Spiritual History

F	Believes in God, reads the Bible regularly, thinks that if you "live a good life according to the Bible, then things will go well for you."
I	Relationship with God is important but going to church is less important.
C	Belongs to a nondenominational Christian church, was raised Baptist, used to go to church regularly, not so much lately.
A	Psychiatry consult, encourage patient to resume medications, chaplain referral in the ED and then referral to pastoral counselor as outpatient, support and continued presence. Ask Eric if the church community could be a place of support for him and, if so, encourage him to reach out to them.

Intervention

Demoralization, defined as lack of meaning, can present as depression. Meaninglessness can be so intense as to provoke desperate thoughts such as suicide. Furthermore, patients who are demoralized may stop taking medications, thinking the medications are of no use. This can further complicate depression. Working with patients on the issues of meaning can be therapeutic. In this case, the intervention would address both emotional and spiritual suffering and referrals to both mental health and spiritual care professionals would be indicated. Continued presence and support would be essential on the part of all health care professionals working with Eric. Finally, asking whether the spiritual community could be of support would also be important.

Case 8: "God Is Punishing Me"

Ms. Lopez is a fifty-eight-year-old female with a history of multiple sclerosis, diagnosed when she was twenty years old in her native country, Brazil. Her disease has been quiescent for the most part and she always attributed this to her strong faith and positive mental attitude. She has no other medical problems except for well-controlled hypertension and arthritis in her left knee.

Ms. Lopez is now in the hospital following surgery for left knee replacement. The surgery went well, but the orthopedists are concerned since the blood pressure has been more difficult to control postoperatively. They also note that in physical therapy she is in a lot of pain but is not taking enough pain meds, thus affecting her ability to participate in physical therapy. They ask the pain team to consult with the patient.

The nurse on the team comes to evaluate Ms. Lopez and as part of the whole history obtains a spiritual history. During the spiritual history, Ms. Lopez reveals that family is important to her. She starts crying and mentions that her son is dying of AIDS and her other son has just failed his courses at college. She exclaims, "I must have done something so bad that God is punishing my children for my sins."

Spiritual History

F	Catholic, active in her church. Meaning stems from her relationship with God, her family, and her work (she feels her work in doing refugee aid makes a difference in people's lives).
I	Her religious and spiritual values impact her lifestyle. Her faith has helped her cope with divorce, problems with her children, and with life in general.
C	She is active in her church and attends a meditation class weekly. She sees a spiritual director at her church.
A	Presence, referral to chaplain, referral to social work for arranging a family meeting, referral to support group for single mothers, encourage continuing work with spiritual director at church.

Intervention

People can interpret their situation through many narratives. Religious beliefs can be the expression of deep suffering. In Ms. Lopez's case, she expresses her deep pain regarding her children's situation as a failing on her part. She prides herself in being a good mother and a religious woman who believes in the goodness of God. Her way of reconciling those aspects of herself is to blame herself for her children's suffering rather than be angry at God or disappointed in her children. In her current clinical situation, she feels powerless over everything around her—her children, her health. Her only control is over the medication and whether she will participate in therapy. Referral to a chaplain and help Ms Lopez examine her beliefs as well as her relationships with God and with her children would be indicated. Helping her share some of her concerns with her children may also help her.

The plan would therefore be a chaplain referral, social work referral for a family meeting, and for a recommendation about a support groups as an outpatient. Once she is discharged, the plan is to continue working with her spiritual director.

Case 9: Chief Concern

Mr. Ben Culver is a fifty-five-year-old male who has just found out that he is diagnosed with a chief complaint of new onset NIDDM. Ben becomes despondent after the doctor tells him of his diagnosis. The doctor probes deeper about the patient's concerns. Ben tells the doctor his uncle died of complications from diabetes, including BKA and ESRD, requiring dialysis. He is fearful this will happen to him. The physician explores his fear and asks if he has any spiritual beliefs that might help him.

Spiritual History

F	Presbyterian, meaning is doing good in his life and helping others.
I	Relationship with God helps . . . everything happens for a reason and God has his reasons. Belief in God has helped him overcome fear before.
C	Church community is helpful to Ben. There are support groups there for people who are ill. There is also a faith community nurse that runs some health programs at the church.
A	Patient interested in going to the support group at his church and also working with the faith community nurse at the church.

Intervention

People understand diagnosis based on their own experience or that of family and friends. These narratives can profoundly affect how a patient copes with his or her diagnosis. Spiritual or religious beliefs can impact how someone copes with illness. Faith communities may have faith community nurses that work at the churches. Linking patients with resources at their churches can be very beneficial to the patient.

This case also demonstrates the importance of recognizing that the important issues for patients, i.e., their chief concerns may be deeper than the "chief complaints." Ben's chief complaint listed on the chart was a newly diagnosed case of diabetes. His chief concern, however, was his understanding of his diagnosis. It is important for clinicians to discuss both the chief complaint and concern.

The plan would be to encourage patient to attend the support groups at his church, work with the faith community nurse, and continue to listen and be present with Mr. Culver about his concerns.

Case 10: Nature as Spirituality

Ms. Betty Smith is a fifty-two-year-old female with a breast mass. She has a strong family history of breast cancer. Her mother died of breast cancer when the patient was eighteen years old. Her two sisters have breast cancer.

Spiritual History

F	Meaning is in nature
I	"I feel at one with nature. Each morning I sit on my patio looking out over the trees in the woods and feel 'centered and with purpose.'" "This is so important to me that if I am dying I would want to be in a hospice that has nature around it. Please write that in my chart."
C	Close friends show share beliefs and values. They hike together and do rituals that have a Native American origin.
A	After the discussion about belief, she still tries to meditate, focusing on nature, on a daily basis to increase her peacefulness and her ability to cope with whatever the biopsy shows.

Intervention

In this case, the role of nature is very important to Ms. Smith. She is also interested in learning more about meditation to help her cope. Thus, her plan would be to respect her beliefs, offer her presence, note her beliefs in the chart and how it would impact her choice of where she dies, and refer her for meditation classes.

Case 11: Religious Rituals and Practices

Rana is a twenty-four-year-old female who is three months pregnant. She has been feeling lightheaded the last few days.

Spiritual History

F	Muslim, Allah gives meaning to her.
I	Very important, prays five times daily, adheres to all practices, is fasting now with Ramadan, which started five days ago.
C	Mosque community and family. Listens to husband and imam in all matters. Is aware she may not need to fast but would like to talk with imam to get permission.
A	Encourage patient to talk with imam about rules for pregnant women during Ramadan; invite patient to ask imam to come to next office visit if she would like, encourage her to take in appropriate fluids and po intake.

Intervention

Some religious and cultural practices can have a negative outcome on health. In this case, fasting has caused this patient to be lightheaded and dehydrated. While her religion exempts her from the fast, she needs to hear that from an imam. People may not always be aware of the rules of certain rituals and practices of their religion and may need clarification from their religious leaders. The plan should include respecting the beliefs and practices and helping the patient get clarification with her religious leader about the observance in light of her health issues.

Case 12: The Case of Miracles

Mrs. M. is a seventy-two-year-old female with COPD, on mechanical ventilator for two months because of ARDS and MOSF. Doctors believe Mrs. M. may have only a 1 percent chance of being extubated successfully. They have discussions with family about limiting life-sustaining interventions. Mrs. M. has an advance directive that indicates her husband should be her surrogate but does not provide specifics as to the care she would want. Mr. M. and the two children insist that mechanical ventilation should be continued.

Spiritual History (of the Husband)

F	Baptist, God is meaning and "he is the only one who can make life and death decisions." "We will not let you turn off the machine."
I	Faith is central to husband's and wife's life and decision making, prayer is key to their survival and well-being, strong belief in miracles.
C	Husband and wife are both active church members; great support from church.
A	Presence, referral to chaplain, invite family's pastor to hospital if desired by family, encourage rituals around bedside.

Intervention

- Listen to family's belief in miracles and to their religious/spiritual beliefs
- Find common ground ("I wish, I hope, What do you believe in")
- Explore whether the religious beliefs have other implications for patient's care
- Ask patient's family about other hopes for the patient. (Do not ask initially, as that may seem dismissive of the family's religious beliefs.)
- Work with chaplains, clergy, religious leaders

Plan is for the medical team to be open and respectful to Mr. M.'s beliefs yet honest about the prognosis from the biomedical perspective. Align with the family by acknowledging hope and wishes. Refer to chaplain to help family explore their wishes and beliefs further.

Appendix E Professional Chaplaincy

Qualifications of Professional Chaplaincy (QUA)

The candidate for certification must:

QUA1: Provide documentation of current endorsement or of good standing in accordance with the requirements of his/her own faith tradition.

QUA2: Be current in the payment of the professional association's annual dues.

QUA3: Have completed an undergraduate degree from a college, university, or theological school accredited by a member of the Council for Higher Education Accreditation (www.chea.org); and a graduate-level theological degree from a college, university, or theological school accredited by a member of the Council for Higher Education Accreditation. Equivalencies for the undergraduate and/or graduate level theological degree will be granted by the individual professional organizations according to their own established guidelines.

QUA4: Provide documentation of a minimum of four units of Clinical Pastoral Education (CPE) accredited by the Association for Clinical Pastoral Education (ACPE), the United States Conference of Catholic Bishops Commission on Certification and Accreditation, or the Canadian Association for Pastoral Practice and Education (CAPPE/ACPEP). Equivalency for one unit of CPE may be considered.

Section I: Theory of Pastoral Care (TPC)

The candidate for certification will demonstrate the ability to:

TPC1: Articulate a theology of spiritual care that is integrated with a theory of pastoral practice.

TPC2: Incorporate a working knowledge of psychological and sociological disciplines and religious beliefs and practices in the provision of pastoral care.

TPC3: Incorporate the spiritual and emotional dimensions of human development into the practice of pastoral care.

TPC4: Incorporate a working knowledge of ethics appropriate to the pastoral context.

TPC5: Articulate a conc TPC4: Incorporate a working knowledge of ethics appropriate to the pastoral context.

Section II: Identity and Conduct (IDC)

The candidate for certification will demonstrate the ability to:

IDC1: Function pastorally in a manner that respects the physical, emotional, and spiritual boundaries of others.

IDC2: Use pastoral authority appropriately.

IDC3: Identify one's professional strengths and limitations in the provision of pastoral care.

IDC4: Articulate ways in which one's feelings, attitudes, values, and assumptions affect one's pastoral care.

IDC5: Advocate for the persons in one's care.

IDC6: Function within the Common Code of Ethics for Chaplains, Pastoral Counselors, Pastoral Educators, and Students.

IDC7: Attend to one's own physical, emotional, and spiritual well-being.

IDC8: Communicate effectively orally and in writing.

IDC9: Present oneself in a manner that reflects professional behavior, including appropriate attire and personal hygiene.

Section III: Pastoral (PAS)

The candidate for certification will demonstrate the ability to:

PAS1: Establish, deepen, and end pastoral relationships with sensitivity, openness, and respect.

PAS2: Provide effective pastoral support that contributes to well-being of patients, their families, and staff.

PAS3: Provide pastoral care that respects diversity and differences including, but not limited to, culture, gender, sexual orientation, and spiritual/religious practices.

PAS4: Triage and manage crises in the practice of pastoral care.

PAS5: Provide pastoral care to persons experiencing loss and grief.

PAS6: Formulate and utilize spiritual assessments in order to contribute to plans of care.

PAS7: Provide religious/spiritual resources appropriate to the care of patients, families, and staff.

PAS8: Develop, coordinate, and facilitate public worship/spiritual practices appropriate to diverse settings and needs.

PAS9: Facilitate theological reflection in the practice of pastoral care.

Section IV: Professional (PRO)

The candidate for certification will demonstrate the ability to:

PRO1: Promote the integration of pastoral/spiritual care into the life and service of the institution in which it resides.

PRO2: Establish and maintain professional and interdisciplinary relationships.

PRO3: Articulate an understanding of institutional culture and systems, and systemic relationships.

PRO4: Support, promote, and encourage ethical decision making and care.

PRO5: Document one's contribution of care effectively in the appropriate records.

PRO6: Foster a collaborative relationship with community clergy and faith group leaders.

Requirements for the Maintenance (MNT) of Certification

In order to maintain status as a certified chaplain, the chaplain must:

MNT1: Participate in a peer review process every fifth year.

MNT2: Document fifty (50) hours of annual continuing education. (Recommendation that personal therapy, spiritual direction, supervision, and/or peer review be acceptable options for continuing education hours.)

MNT3: Provide documentation every fifth year of current endorsement or of good standing in accordance with the requirements of his/her own faith tradition.

MNT4: Be current in the payment of the professional association's annual dues.

MNT5: Adhere to the Common Code of Ethics for Chaplains, Pastoral Counselors, Pastoral Educators, and Students.

(Spiritual Care Collaborative Standards, 2007)

Appendix F   Listing of Research Instruments

Quality of Life Scale/Cancer Patient/Cancer Survivor

Ferrell, B. R., Dow, K. H., & Grant, M. (1995). Measurements of the quality of life in cancer survivors. *Quality of Life Research, 4*, 523–531.

Age Universal I-E Scale

Gorsuch, R. L., & Venable, G. D. (1983). Development of an "age universal" I-E scale. *Journal for the Scientific Study of Religion, 22*(2), 181–187.

Sacred Loss and Desecration Scale

Warner, H. (2009). Generational curse? Spiritual appraisals, spiritual struggles and risk factors for the intergenerational transmission of divorce (PhD, Bowling Green State University, Bowling Green, OH).

Religious Problem-Solving Scale

Pargament, K. I., Kennell, J., Hathaway, W., Grevengoed, N., Newman, J., & Jones, W. (1988). Religion and the problem-solving process: Three styles of coping. *Journal for the Scientific Study of Religion, 27*(1), 90–104.

Negative RCOPE Scale

Pargament, K. I., Koenig, H. G., & Perez, L. M. (2000). The many methods of religious coping: Development and initial validation of the RCOPE. *Journal of Clinical Psychology, 56*(4), 519–543.

Religious Strain Scale

Exline, J. J., Yali, A. M., & Sanderson, W. C. (2000). Guilt, discord, and alienation: The role of religious strain in depression and suicidality. *Journal of Clinical Psychology, 56*(12), 1481–1496.

Religious Doubts Scale

Altemeyer, B. (1989). *Enemies of freedom: Understanding right-wing authoritarianism.* San Francisco: Jossey-Bass.

Spiritual Transformation Scale

Cole, B. S., Hopkins, C. M., Tisak, J., Steel, J. L., & Carr, B. I. (2008). Assessing spiritual growth and spiritual decline following a diagnosis of cancer: Reliability and validity of the spiritual transformation scale. *Psycho-Oncology, 17*(2), 112–121.

Penn Inventory of Scrupulosity

Abramowitz, J. S., Huppert, J. D., Cohen, A. B., Tolin, D. F., & Cahill, S. P. (2002). Religious obsessions and compulsions in a non-clinical sample: The Penn Inventory of Scrupulosity (PIOS). *Behaviour Research and Therapy, 40*(7), 825–838.

Spiritual Support Scale

Maton, K. I. (1989). The stress-buffering role of spiritual support: Cross-sectional and prospective investigations. *Journal for the Scientific Study of Religion, 28*(3), 310–323.

Religious Well-Being Scale

Paloutzian, R. F., Ellison, C. W., Peplau, L. A., & Perlman, D. (1982). *Loneliness: A sourcebook of current theory, research and therapy.* New York: Wiley.

Spirituality Integrated Psychotherapy

Pargament, K. I. (2007). *Spiritually integrated psychotherapy.* New York: Guilford Press.

Brief Serenity Scale

Kreitzer, M. J., Gross, C. R., Waleekhachonloet, O. A., Reilly-Spong, M., & Byrd, M. (2009). The brief serenity scale: A psychometric analysis of a measure of spirituality and well-being. *Journal of Holistic Nursing: Official Journal of the American Holistic Nurses' Association, 27*(1), 7–16.

McGill Quality of Life

Cohen, S. R., Mount, B. M., Strobel, M. G., & Bui, F. (1995). The McGill quality of life questionnaire: A measure of quality of life appropriate for people with advanced disease. A preliminary study of validity and acceptability. *Palliative Medicine, 9*(3), 207–219.

FACIT-Spiritual Well-Being Scale

Peterman, A. H., Fitchett, G., Brady, M. J., Hernandez, L., & Cella, D. (2002). Measuring spiritual well-being in people with cancer: The functional assessment of chronic illness therapy—Spiritual Well-being Scale (FACIT-sp). *Annals of Behavioral Medicine, 24*(1), 49–58.

Duke Religious Index

Sherman, A. C., Plante, T. G., Simonton, S., Adams, D. C., Harbison, C., & Burris, S. K. (2000). A multidimensional measure of religious involvement for cancer patients: The Duke Religious Index. *Supportive Care in Cancer, 8*(2), 102–109.

Positive RCOPE

Pargament, K. I., Koenig, H. G., & Perez, L. M. (2000). The many methods of religious coping: Development and initial validation of the RCOPE. *Journal of Clinical Psychology, 56*(4), 519–543.

Systems of Belief Inventory

Holland, J. C., Kash, K. M., Passik, S., Gronert, M. K., Sison, A., Lederberg, M., Russak, S.M., Baider, L., & Fox, B. (1998). A brief spiritual beliefs inventory for use in quality of life research in life-threatening illness. *Psycho-Oncology, 7*(6), 460–469.

Meaning in Life Scale

Jim, H. S., Purnell, J. Q., Richardson, S. A., Golden-Kreutz, D., & Andersen, B. L. (2006). Measuring meaning in life following cancer. *Quality of Life Research, 15*(8), 1355–1371.

Spiritual Needs Inventory

Hermann, C. P. (2006). Development and testing of the spiritual needs inventory for patients near the end of life. *Oncology Nursing Forum, 33*(4), 737–744.

Spiritual Needs Related to Illness Tool

Taylor, E. J. (2006). Prevalence and associated factors of spiritual needs among patients with cancer and family caregivers. *Oncology Nursing Forum, 33*(4), 729–735.

Beliefs and Values Scale

King, M., Jones, L., Barnes, K., Low, J., Walker, C., Wilkinson, S., Mason,

C., Sutherland, J., & Rookman, A. (2006). Measuring spiritual belief: Development and standardization of a beliefs and values scale. *Psychological Medicine, 36*(3), 417–425.

WHOQOL Spirituality, Religiousness and Personal Beliefs Field-Test Instrument

Mental Health: Evidence & Research, Department of Mental Health & Substance Dependence, World Health Organization. (2002). WHOQOL spirituality, religiousness and personal beliefs (SRPB) field-test instrument: The WHOQOL-100 QUESTIONS PLUS 32 SRPB QUESTIONS. Geneva, Switzerland: World Health Organization. Retrieved March 31, 2009, from http://www.who.int/mental_health/media/en/622.pdf.

Spiritual Involvement and Beliefs Scale

Hatch, R. L., Burg, M. A., Naberhaus, D. S., & Hellmich, L. K. (1998). The Spiritual Involvement and Beliefs Scale: Development and testing of a new instrument. *Journal of Family Practice, 46*(6), 476–486.

Hays, J. C., Meador, K. G., Branch, P. S., & George, L. K. (2001). The Spiritual History Scale in four dimensions (SHS-4): Validity and reliability. *Gerontologist, 41*(2), 239–249.

The Royal Free Questionnaire for Spiritual and Religious Beliefs

King, M., Speck, P., & Thomas, A. (2001). The royal free interview for spiritual and religious beliefs: Development and validation of a self-report version. *Psychological Medicine, 31*(6), 1015–1023.

JAREL Spiritual Well-Being Scale

Hungelmann, J., Kenkel-Rossi, E., Klassen, L., & Stollenwerk, R. (1996). Focus on spiritual well-being: Harmonious interconnectedness of mind-body-spirit—use of the JAREL Spiritual Well-Being Scale. *Geriatric Nursing (New York, N.Y.), 17*(6), 262–266.

Lourdes Medical Center of Burlington County

Survey
Lourdes Medical Center of Burlington County
218 Sunset Road, Willingboro, NJ 08046; 609-835-2900

Appendix G   Listing of Curricula in Spirituality and Health

GWish Competencies and Learning Objectives for Spirituality and Health Education

www.gwish.org

Medical School Objectives Project

Association of American Medical Colleges. (1999). *Report III: Contemporary issues in medicine: Communication in medicine: Medical school objectives project.* Washington, DC: AAMC. Retrieved from https://services.aamc.org/Publications/showfile .cfm?file=version89.pdf&prd_id=200&prv_id=241&pdf_id=89

Spirituality and Health Orientation Curriculum

Kreslins, D. (2009). *The spirituality and health orientation curriculum.* Grand Rapids, MI: Saint Mary's Health Care.

DSM-IV Religious and Spiritual Problems

Lukoff, D. (2005). *DSM-IV religious and spiritual problems.* Retrieved November 18, 2009, from http://www.virtualcs.com/dsm4/course _dsmiv.asp.

Spiritual and Religious Care Competencies for Specialist Palliative Care

Marie Curie Cancer Care. (n.d.). Spiritual and religious care competencies for specialist palliative care. London: Marie Curie Cancer Care. Retrieved from http://www.mariecurie.org.uk/ forhealthcareprofessionals/spiritualandreligiouscare/index.htm.

Appendix H Spirituality Centers and Other Relevant Websites

Spirituality Centers:

Association for Spirituality and Mental Health
Department of Psychiatry of the University of Ottawa and the Ontario
    Multifaith Council on Spiritual and Religious Care
Ottawa, Canada
Year Started: 2007
http://www.spiritualityandmentalhealth.org

Benson-Henry Institute for Mind Body Medicine
Massachusetts General Hospital
http://www.massgeneral.org/bhi/

Canadian Research Institute of Spirituality and Healing
Vancouver, Canada
Year Started: 2006
http://www.crish.org/index.html

Center for Spirituality and Healing
University of Minnesota
Year Started: 1995
http://www.csh.umn.edu/

Center for Spirituality and Health
University of Florida
Year Started: 2001
http://www.spiritualityandhealth.ufl.edu/

Centre for Spirituality, Health, and Disability
University of Aberdeen
Aberdeen, Scotland
Year Started: 2006
http://www.abdn.ac.uk/cshad/

Center for the Study of Health, Religion, and Spirituality
Indiana State University
Year Started: 2003
http://web.indstate.edu/psychology/cshrs/

Duke Center for Spirituality, Theology, and Health
Duke University
Year Started: 2007
http://www.spiritualityandhealth.duke.edu/index.html

GWish: The George Washington Institute for Spirituality and Health
George Washington University Medical Center
Year Started: 2001
www.gwish.org

Institute for Spirituality and Health
Palmetto Health
California
http://www.palmettohealth.org/body.cfm?id=1854&oTopID=1

Institute for Spirituality and Health
Texas Medical Center
Year Started: 1955
http://www.ish-tmc.org/index.php

Research Institute for Spirituality and Health
Langenthal, Switzerland
Year Started: 2005
http://www.rish.ch/

The SHIM Institute
Utah
Year Started: 2003
http://www.theshiminstitute.org/

Society for Spirituality, Theology, and Health
Funded in part by a grant from the John Templeton Foundation, affiliated
    with Duke Center
Year Started: 2009
http://www.societysth.org

Spirituality and Health Institute (SHI)
Santa Clara University
http://www.scu.edu/ecppm/shi/index.cfm

Wayne E. Oates Institute
Kentucky
Year Started: 1993
http://www.oates.org/

Other Relevant Websites:

American Association of Pastoral Counselors (AAPC): www.aapc.org

Association for Clinical Pastoral Education (ACPE): www.acpe.edu

Association of Professional Chaplains: www.professionalchaplains.org

City of Hope: http://prc.coh.org

Duke Institute on Care at the End of Life: www.iceol.duke.edu/

The Interfaith Alliance Foundation: www.interfaithalliance.org/home

John Templeton Foundation: www.templeton.org

National Association of Catholic Chaplains (NACC): www.nacc.org

National Association of Jewish Chaplains (NAJC): www.najc.org

Spiritual Care Collaborative: www.spiritualcarecollaborative.org

The U.S. Conference of Catholic Bishops: www.usccb.org

References

Abramson, J. S., & Mizrahi, T. (2003). Understanding collaboration between social workers and physicians: Application of a typology. *Social Work in Healthcare, 37*(2), 71–100.

Ader, R., Cohen, N., & Felten, D. (1995). Psychoneuroimmunology: Interactions between the nervous system and the immune system. *Lancet, 345*(8942), 99–103.

American Academy of Physician Assistants. (2008). *Guidelines for ethical conduct for the physician assistant profession.* Retrieved March 24, 2009, from http://www.aapa.org/images/stories/documents/about_aapa/policymanual/19-EthicalConduct.pdf

American Association of Colleges of Nursing (AACN). (2008).*The essentials of baccalaureate education for professional nursing practice.* Retrieved February 12, 2009, from http://www.aacn.nche.edu/education/pdf/BaccEssentials08.pdf.

American Association of Pastoral Counselors. (n.d.). *What is pastoral counseling?* Retrieved March 31, 2009, from http://www.aapc.org/node/3.

American College of Physicians (ACP). (2009). Position Paper: Ethics Manual. Retrieved August 25, 2009, from http://www.acponline.org/.

American Medical Association. (2001). *Code of medical ethics.* Chicago, IL: American Medical Association. Retrieved November 30, 2009, from http://www.ama-assn.org/ama/pub/physician-resources/medical-ethics/code-medical-ethics/principles-medical-ethics.shtml

American Nurses Association (ANA). (2001). *Code of ethics for nurses with interpretive statement.* Retrieved December 10, 2008, from http://nursingworld.org/MainMenuCategories/ThePracticeofProfessionalNursing/EthicsStandards/CodeofEthics.aspx

American Nurses Association. (2003). *Nursing's social policy statement* (2nd ed.). Silver Spring, MD: American Nurses Association.

American Nurses Association (ANA), & Health Ministries Association (HMA). (2005). *Faith and community nursing: Scope and standards of practice.* Silver Spring, MD: American Nurses Association.

American Psychiatric Association. (2000). *Diagnostic and statistical manual of mental disorders: DSM-IV-TR.* Washington, DC: American Psychiatric Association.

American Psychological Association. (2002). *Ethical principles of psychologists and code of conduct.* Retrieved April 1, 2009, from http://www.apa.org/ethics/code2002.html

American Psychological Association Online. (2001). *End-of-life issues and care.* Retrieved March 15, 2009, from http://www.apa.org/pi/eol/activities.html

Anandarajah, G., & Hight, E. (2001). Spirituality and medical practice: Using the HOPE questions as a practical tool for spiritual assessment. *American Family Physician, 63*(1), 81–89.

Ando, M., Morita, T., Okamoto, T., & Ninosaka, Y. (2008). One-week short-term life review interview can improve spiritual well-being of terminally ill cancer patients. *Psycho-Oncology, 17*(9), 885–890.

Association of American Medical Colleges (AAMC). (1998). *Report I: Learning objectives for medical student education: Guidelines for medical schools.* Washington, DC: AAMC. Retrieved March 31, 2009, from https://services.aamc.org/Publications/showfile.cfm?file=version87.pdf&prd_id=198&prv_id=239&pdf_id=87

Association of American Medical Colleges (AAMC). (1999). *Report III: Contemporary issues in medicine: Communication in Medicine.* Washington, DC: AAMC. Retrieved March 31, 2009, from https://services.aamc.org/Publications/showfile.cfm?file=version89.pdf&prd_id=200&prv_id=241&pdf_id=89

Astrow, A. B., Puchalski, C. M., & Sulmasy, D. P. (2001). Religion, spirituality, and healthcare: Social, ethical, and practical considerations. *American Journal of Medicine, 110*(4), 283–287.

Balboni, T. A., Vanderwerker, L., Block, S. D., Paulk, M. E., Lathan, C. S., Peteet, J. R., Prigerson, H. G. (2007). Religiousness and spiritual support among advanced cancer patients and associations with end-of-life treatment preferences and quality of life. *Journal of Clinical Oncology, 25*(5), 555–560.

Balducci, L. (2008). And a time to die (E un tempo per morire). *Journal of Medicine and the Person, 6*(3), 99–103.

Barbour, I. G. (1990). *Religion in an age of science: The Gifford Lectures, 1989–1991* (vol. 1). San Francisco: Harper & Row.

Barnes, P., Powell-Griner, E., McFann, K., & Nahin, R. (2002). Complementary and alternative medicine use among adults: United States. *CDC Advance Data Report #343*. Retrieved March 31, 2009, from http://www.cdc.gov/nchs/data/ad/ad343.pdf

Barnum, B. S. (1996). *Spirituality in nursing: From traditional to new age.* New York: Springer Publishing.

Bengtson, V. L., & Schaie, K. W. (1999). *Handbook of theories of aging.* New York: Springer Publishing Company.

Benson, H. (1996). *Timeless healing: The power and biology of belief.* New York: Simon & Schuster.

Benson, H., & Proctor, W. (1984). *Beyond the relaxation response: How to harness the healing power of your personal beliefs.* New York: Times Books.

Bergin, A. E. (1991). Values and religious issues in psychotherapy and mental health. *American Psychologist, 46*(4), 394–403.

Bergin, A. E., & Strupp, H. H. (1972). *Changing frontiers in the science of psychotherapy.* Chicago: Aldine-Atherton.

Bolen, J. S. (1996). *Close to the bone: Life-threatening illness and the search for meaning.* New York: Touchstone.

Boscaglia, N., Clarke, D. M., Jobling, T. W., & Quinn, M. A. (2005). The contribution of spirituality and spiritual coping to anxiety and depression in women with a recent diagnosis of gynecological cancer. *International Journal of Gynecological Cancer, 15*(5), 755–761.

Borneman, T., Puchalski, C. & Ferrell, B. (In press). Evaluation of the FICA tool for spiritual assessment. *Journal of Pain and Symptom Management.*

Bradshaw, J. (1988). *Bradshaw on: The family.* Deerfield Beach, FL: Health Communications.

Breitbart, W. (2003). Reframing hope: Meaning-centered care for patients near the end of life. Interview by Karen S. Heller. *Journal of Palliative Medicine, 6*(6), 979–988.

Breitbart, W., Kissane, D., & Chochinov, H. M. (2009). Dignity, meaning and demoralization: Emerging paradigms in end of life care. In H. M. Chochinov & W. Breitbart (Eds.), *Handbook of Psychiatry in Palliative Medicine* (pp. 324–340). New York: Oxford University Press.

Breitbart, W., Rosenfeld, B. D., & Passik, S. D. (1996). Interest in physician-assisted suicide among ambulatory HIV-infected patients. *American Journal of Psychiatry, 153*(2), 238–242.

Bridges, W. (2004). *Transitions: Making sense of life's changes.* New York: DaCapo Press.

Brunnhuber, K., Nash, S., Meier, D. E., Weissman, D. E., & Woodcock. J. (2008). *Putting evidence into practice: Palliative care.* London: BMJ Publishing Group.

Bryant, S. (2005). *Compassionate medicine interview responses.* Retrieved December 10, 2008, from http://www.stolaf.edu/depts/cis/wp/bryant/responses.htm

Bryson, K. A. (2004). Spirituality, meaning, and transcendence. *Palliative & Supportive Care, 2*(3), 321–328.

Buber, M. (1958). *I and Thou.* New York: Scribner.

Burgener, S. C. (1999). Predicting quality of life in caregivers of Alzheimer's patients: The role of support from and involvement with the religious community. *Journal of Pastoral Care, 53*(4), 433–446.

Burke, K. (2006). Religion, spirituality and health. In: S. Gehlert &

T. E. Browne (Eds.), *The handbook of health and social work.* (pp. 282–304). Hoboken, NJ: John Wiley & Sons.

Burkhardt, M. A., & Nagai-Jacobson, M. (2000). Spirituality and health. In B. M. Dossey, L. Keegan, & C. E. Guzetaa (Eds.), *Holistic nursing: A handbook for practice* (3rd ed., pp. 91–121). Gaithersburg, MD: Aspen.

Canda, E., & Furman, L. (1999). *Spiritual diversity in social work practice: The heart of helping.* New York: Free Press.

Canda, E., & Smith, E. D. (Eds.). (2001). *Transpersonal perspective on spirituality in social work.* New York: Haworth Press.

Canadian Association for Pastoral Practice and Education (CAPPE/ACPEP). (2008). *CAPPE/ACPEP code of ethics for chaplains, pastoral counselors, pastors, pastoral educators and students.* Retrieved March 31, 2009, from http://www.cappe.org/resources/code_of_ethics/CAPPE-ACPEP%20Code%20of%20Ethics%20revised%20April%202008.pdf

Cassell, E. J. (1982). The nature of suffering and the goals of medicine. *New England Journal of Medicine, 306*(11), 639–645.

Cassell, E. J. (1991). *The nature of suffering and the goals of medicine.* New York: Oxford University Press.

CBS News/New York Times Poll. (1998, April 29). Retrieved April 1, 2009, from http://poll.orspub.com/document.php?id=quest98.out_24099&type=hitlist&num=0

Chao, C. S., Chen, C. H., & Yen, M. (2002). The essence of spirituality of terminally ill patients. *Journal of Nursing Research: JNR, 10*(4), 237–245.

Chochinov, H. M. (2002). Dignity-conserving care—a new model for palliative care: Helping the patient feel valued. *Journal of the American Medical Association, 287*(17), 2253–2260.

Chochinov, H. M. (2006). Dying, dignity, and new horizons in palliative end-of-life care. *CA: A Cancer Journal for Clinicians, 56*(2), 84–103.

Chochinov, H. M., & Breitbart, W. (2009). *Handbook of Psychiatry in Palliative Medicine.* New York: Oxford University Press.

Chochinov, H. M., Hack, T., Hassard, T., Kristjanson, L .J., McClement, S., & Harlos, M. (2004). Dignity and psychotherapeutic considerations in end-of-life care. *Journal of Palliative Care, 20*(3), 134–142.

Chochinov, H. M., Hack, T., McClement, S., Kristjanson, L., & Harlos, M. (2002). Dignity in the terminally ill: A developing empirical model. *Social Science & Medicine, 54*(3), 433–443.

Chow, E. O., & Nelson-Becker, H. (in press). Spiritual distress to spiritual transformation: Stroke survivor narratives from Hong Kong. *Journal of Aging Studies, 25*(1).

Clark, C. C., Cross, J. R., Deane, D. M., & Lowry, L. W. (1991). Spirituality: Integral to quality care. *Holistic Nursing Practice, 5*(3), 67–76.

Clarke, J. (2006). A discussion paper about "meaning" in the nursing literature on spirituality: An interpretation of meaning as "ultimate concern" using the work of Paul Tillich. *International Journal of Nursing Studies, 43*(7), 915–921.

Cohen, S. R., & Leis, A. (2002). What determines the quality of life of terminally ill cancer patients from their own perspective? *Journal of Palliative Care, 18*(1), 48–58.

Cohen, S. R., Mount, B. M., Strobel, M. G., & Bui, F. (1995). The McGill quality of life questionnaire: A measure of quality of life appropriate for people with advanced disease. A preliminary study of validity and acceptability. *Palliative Medicine, 9*(3), 207–219.

Cohen, S. R., Mount, B. M., Tomas, J. J., & Mount, L. F. (1996). Existential well-being is an important determinant of quality of life: Evidence from the McGill quality of life questionnaire. *Cancer, 77*(3), 576–586.

Cole, B., Hopkins, C., Tisak, J., Steel, J., & Carr, B. (2007). Assessing spiritual growth and spiritual decline following a diagnosis of cancer: Reliability and validity of the spiritual transformation scale. *Psycho-Oncology, 17*(2), 112–121.

Compassion. (2008). In *Oxford English dictionary: The definitive record of the English language.* Retrieved December 10, 2008, from http://oed.com.

Congress, E. P. (2004). Cultural and ethical issues in working with culturally diverse patients and their families: The use of the culturagram to promote cultural competent practice in healthcare settings. *Social Work in Healthcare, 39*(3–4), 249–262.

Cotton, S., Puchalski, C. M., Sherman, S. N., Mrus, J. M., Peterman, A. H., Feinberg, J., Pargament, K. I., Justice, A. C., Leonard, A. C., Tsevat, J. (2006). Spirituality and religion in patients with HIV/AIDS. *Journal of General Internal Medicine, 21*(Suppl 5), S5–13.

Cousineau, N., McDowell, I., Hotz, S., & Hebert, P. (2003). Measuring chronic patients' feelings of being a burden to their caregivers: Development and preliminary validation of a scale. *Medical Care, 41*(1), 110–118.

Curtsinger, G., & Pierini, P. (1991). *The spiritual canticle of St. John of the Cross.* Manfield, TX: Latitudes.

Cutshall, S., & Miller, J. (2001). *The art of being a healing presence.* Fort Wayne, IN: Willowgreen.

Daaelman, T. P., & Hanson, L. C. (2008). An exploratory study of spiritual care at the end of life. *Annals of Family Medicine, 6*(5), 406–411.

Dalai Lama, Cutler, H. C., & Gardner, G. (1998). *The art of happiness: A handbook for living.* New York: Riverbend.

de Figueiredo, J. M. (1993). Depression and demoralization: Phenomenologic differences and research perspectives. *Comprehensive Psychiatry, 34*(5), 308–311.

Despair. (2009). In *Merriam-Webster online dictionary*. Retrieved [date] from http://www.merriam-webster.com/dictionary

Dignity. (2009). In *Merriam-Webster online dictionary*. Retrieved from http://www.merriam-webster.com/dictionary.

Doka, K. J. (2008). *Counseling individuals with life-threatening illness*. New York: Springer Publishing Company.

Duffy, J. Personal communication.

Dunevitz, B. (1997). Collaboration—in a variety of ways—creates healthcare value. *Nursing Economics, 15*(4), 218–219.

Edmondson, D., Park, C. L., Chaudoir, S. R., & Wortmann, J. H. (2008). Death without god: Religious struggle, death concerns, and depression in the terminally ill. *Psychological Science, 19*(8), 754–758.

Ehman, J. W., Ott, B. B., Short, T. H., Ciampa, R. C., & Hansen-Flaschen, J. (1999). Do patients want physicians to inquire about their spiritual or religious beliefs if they become gravely ill? *Archives of Internal Medicine, 159*(15), 1803–1806.

Elder, G. H. (2001). Encyclopedia of aging: A comprehensive multidisciplinary review of gerontology and geriatrics. In G. Maddox, R. Atchley, J. Evans, C. E. Finch, R. Kane, & M. Mezey (Eds.), (3rd ed., pp. 593–596). New York: Springer.

Elkins, D. N., Hedstrom, L. J., Hughes, L. L., Leaf, J. A., & Saunders, C. (1988). Toward a humanistic phenomenological spirituality definition, description and measurement. *Journal of Humanistic Psychology, 28*(4), 5–18.

Emblen, J. D. (1992). Religion and spirituality defined according to current use in nursing literature. *Journal of Professional Nursing, 8*(1), 41–47.

End-of-Life Nursing Education Consortium (ELNEC). (2009). End-of-Life Nursing Education Consortium (ELNEC) Fact Sheet. Retrieved August 24, 2009, from www.aacn.nche.edu/ELNEC/factsheet.htm

Engel, G. L. (1977). The need for a new medical model: A challenge for biomedicine. *Science, 196*(4286), 129–136.

Engel, G. L. (1992). How much longer must medicine's science be bound by a seventeenth-century world view? *Psychotherapy and Psychosomatics, 57*(1–2), 3–16.

Epley, N., Savitsky, K., & Gilovich, T. (2002). Empathy neglect: Reconciling the spotlight effect and the correspondence bias. *Journal of Personality & Social Psychology, 83*(2), 300–312.

Evans-Wentz, W. (1927). *The Tibetan Book of the Dead*. (Kazi Dawa Samdup, Trans.). Oxford: Oxford University Press.

Existentialism. (2008). In *Merriam-Webster online*. Retrieved February 10, 2009 from http://www.merriam-webster.com/.

Faith. (2009). In Wikipedia. Retrieved August 21, 2009, from http://en.wikipedia.org.

Ferrell, B. R., & Coyle, N. (2006). *Textbook of palliative nursing* (2nd ed.). New York: Oxford University Press.

Ferrell, B. R., & Coyle, N. (2008). The nature of suffering and the goals of nursing. *Oncology Nursing Forum, 35*(2), 241–247.

Ferris, F. D., von Gunten, C. F., & Emanuel, L. L. (2003). Competency in end-of-life care: Last hours of life. *Journal of Palliative Medicine, 6*(4), 605–613.

Field, M. J., & Cassel, C. K. (1997). *Approaching death: Improving care at the end of life.* Washington, DC: National Academy Press.

Figley, C. R. (1995). *Compassion fatigue: Coping with secondary traumatic stress disorder in those who treat the traumatized.* New York: Brunner/Mazel.

Fitchett, G. (2002). *Assessing spiritual needs: A guide for caregivers.* Lima, OH: Academic Renewal Press..

Fitchett, G., Murphy, P. E., Kim, J., Gibbons, J. L., Cameron, J. R., & Davis, J. A. (2004). Religious struggle: Prevalence, correlates and mental health risks in diabetic, congestive heart failure, and oncology patients. *International Journal of Psychiatry in Medicine, 34*(2), 179–196.

Fitchett, G., & Risk, J. L. (2009). Screening for spiritual struggle. *Journal of Pastoral Care and Counseling,* [online] *63* (1 & 2).

Fitchett, G., & Roberts, P. A. (2003). In the garden with Andrea: Spiritual assessment in end of life care. In C. M. Puchalski (Ed.), *Walking together: Physicians, chaplains and clergy caring for the sick* (pp. 23–31). Washington, DC: George Washington Institute for Spirituality and Health.

Flexner A. (1910). *Medical education in the United States and Canada.* New York: Carnegie Foundation for the Advancement of Teaching.

Foglio, J. P., & Brody, H. (1988). Religion, faith, and family medicine. *Journal of Family Practice, 27*(5), 473–474.

Fowler, J. W. (1995). *Stages of faith: The psychology of human development and the quest for meaning.* San Francisco: Harper & Row.

Frankl, V. E. (1963). *Man's search for meaning.* New York: Washington Square Press, Simon & Schuster.

Galek, K., Flannelly, K. J., Vane, A., & Galek, R. M. (2005). Assessing a patient's spiritual needs: A comprehensive instrument. *Holistic Nursing Practice, 19*(2), 62–69.

Gallup International Institute. (1997). *Spiritual beliefs and the dying process.* Princeton, NJ: Gallup International Institute.

George Washington University & George Washington University Institute for Spirituality and Health (GWish). (2008). Prepared as the final class project for Practical Tools in Spiritual Care, a course in the Online Graduate Certificate Program in Spirituality and Health, C. Puchalski, MD, Course Director.

Gilbert, D. T., & Malone, P. S. (1995). The correspondence bias. *Psychological Bulletin, 117*(1), 21–38.

Gillum, R. F., King, D. E., Obisesan, T. O., & Koenig, H. G. (2008). Frequency of attendance at religious services and mortality in a U.S. national cohort. *Annals of Epidemiology, 18*(2), 124–129.

Griffith, J. L., & Griffith, M. E. (2002). *Encountering the sacred in psychotherapy: How to talk with people about their spiritual lives.* New York: Guilford Press.

Hart, J. (2008). Spirituality and health. *Alternative and Complementary Therapist, 14*(4), 189.

Hauss, C. (2003). "Reconciliation." *Beyond Intractability.* Eds. Guy Burgess and Heidi Burgess. Conflict Research Consortium, University of Colorado, Boulder. Posted: September 2003 http://www. beyondintractability.org/essay/reconciliation/

Hays, J. C., Meador, K. G., Branch, P. S., & George, L. K. (2001). The spiritual history scale in four dimensions (SHS-4): Validity and reliability. *Gerontologist, 41* (2) 239–249. Retrieved from SCOPUS database.

Health Grades, Inc. (2009). *Isolation. Wrong diagnosis.* Retrieved August 21, 2009, from http://www.wrongdiagnosis.com/sym/isolation.htm#intro

Health Insurance Portability and Accountability Act. (1966). HIPAA. Retrieved August 25, 2009, from http://aspe.os.dhhs.gov/admnsimp/ pl104191.htm#Subtitle

Hearnshaw, L. S. (1987). *The shaping of modern psychology.* London: Routledge & Kegan Paul.

Hesse, M. B. (1980). *Revolutions and reconstructions in the philosophy of science.* Bloomington: Indiana University Press.

Hodge, D. R. (2001). Spiritual assessment: A review of major qualitative methods and a new framework for assessing spirituality. *Social Work, 46*(3), 203–214.

Hodges, M., London, M. R., & Lundstedt, J. (2006). Family-driven quality improvement in inpatient end-of-life care. *Journal for Healthcare Quality, 28*(2), 20–26.

Holland, J., & Neimeyer, R. (2005). Reducing the risk of burnout in end-of-life care settings: The role of daily spiritual experiences and training. *Palliative and Supportive Care, 3,* 173–181.

Hooyman, N. R., & Kiyak, H. A. (2005). *Social gerontology: A multidisciplinary perspective* (7th ed.). Boston: Allyn and Bacon.

Hooyman, N. R., & Kramer, B. J. (2006). *Living through loss: Interventions across the life span.* New York: Columbia University Press.

Hope. (2009). In *American heritage dictionary of the English language* (4th ed.). Retrieved August 21, 2009, from http://dictionary.reference.com.

Hungelmann, J., Kenkel-Rossi, E., Klassen, L., & Stollenwerk, R. (1996).

Focus on spiritual well-being: Harmonious interconnectedness of mind-body-spirit use of the JAREL spiritual well-being scale: Assessment of spiritual well-being is essential to the health of individuals. *Geriatric Nursing, 17*(6), 262–266.

Institute for Alternative Futures. (2004). *Patient-centered care 2015: Scenarios, vision, goals and next steps.* Alexandria, VA: Picker Institute. Retrieved from http://www.altfutures.com/pubs/Picker%20 Final%20Report%20May%2014%202004.pdf

Institute of Medicine (Ed.). (2001). *Crossing the quality chasm: A new health system for the 21st century.* Washington, DC: National Academy Press.

International Council of Nurses. (2006). *International Council of Nurses code for nurses.* Geneva, Switzerland: International Council of Nurses. Retrieved December 18, 2008, from http://www.icn.ch/ icncode.pdf

Jaarsma, T. A., Pool, G., Sanderman, R., & Ranchor, A. V. (2006). Psychometric properties of the Dutch version of the posttraumatic growth inventory among cancer patients. *Psycho-Oncology, 15*(10), 911–920.

James, W. (1905). *The varieties of religious experience.* New York: Longmans, Green, and Co.

Jim, H. S., Purnell, J. Q., Richardson, S. A., Golden-Kreutz, D., & Andersen, B. L. (2006). Measuring meaning in life following cancer. *Quality of Life Research, 15*(8), 1355–1371.

Johnson, M., Bulechek, G., Butcher, H., Dochterman, J., Maas, M., Moorhead S., & Swanson, E. (2006). *NANDA, NOC, and NICLinkages, nursing diagnoses, outcomes and interventions.* St. Louis, MO: Mosby.

Joint Commission. (2008). *Spiritual assessment.* Retrieved December 10, 2008, from http://www.jointcommission.org/AccreditationPrograms/ LongTermCare/Standards/09_FAQs/PC/Spiritual_Assessment.htm

Joint Commission on Accreditation of Healthcare Organizations. (1996). *Comprehensive accreditation manual for hospitals: The official handbook.* Oakbrook Terrace, IL: Joint Commission on Accreditation of Healthcare Organizations.

Joint Commission on Accrediting on Health Organizations. (2005). Evaluating your Spiritual Assessment Process. *The Source, 3*(2), 6–7. Retrieved March 31, 2009, from http://www.ingentaconnect.com/ content/jcaho/jcts/2005/00000003/00000002

Joint Commission Resources. (2005). *Providing culturally and linguistically competent health care.* Oakbrook Terrace, IL: Joint Commission Resources.

Jonas, H. (2001). *The phenomenon of life: Towards a philosophical biology.* Evanston, IL: Northwestern University Press.

Kade, W. J. (2000). Death with dignity: A case study. *Annals of Internal Medicine, 132*(6), 504–506.

Kaeton, E. (1998). Pastoral care at the end of life: Listening for the question beneath the question. *Journal of Palliative Medicine, 1*(3), 285–289.

Karier, C. J. (1986). *Scientists of the mind: Intellectual founders of modern psychology.* Urbana: University of Illinois Press.

Kelcourse, F. B. (2004). *Human development and faith: Life-Cycle Stages of body, mind and soul.* St. Louis: Chalice Press.

Kelly, D. (2007). *Applying quality management in healthcare: A systems approach* (2nd ed). Chicago, IL: Health Administration Press.

Kim, M. J., McFarland, G., & McLane, A. (1984). *Classification of nursing diagnosis: Proceedings of the fifth national conference.* St. Louis, MO: Mosby.

King, D. E. (2000). *Faith, spirituality and medicine: Toward the making of a healing practitioner.* Binghamton, NY: Haworth Pastoral Press.

King, D. E., & Bushwick, B. (1994). Beliefs and attitudes of hospital inpatients about faith healing and prayer. *Journal of Family Practice, 39*(4), 349–352.

Kissane, D. W., Clarke, D. M., & Street, A. F. (2001). Demoralization syndrome–a relevant psychiatric diagnosis for palliative care. *Journal of Palliative Care, 17*(1), 12–21.

Ko, E. J. (2008). Advance care planning among Korean American and non-Hispanic white older adults. (Doctoral dissertation, University of Kansas).

Koenig, H. G., McCullough, M. E., & Larson, D. B. (2001). *Handbook of religion and health.* New York: Oxford University Press.

Koenig, H. G., Pargament, K. I., & Nielson, J. (1998). Religious coping and health status in medically ill hospitalized older adults. *The Journal of Nervous and Mental Disease, 186*(9), 513–521.

La Puma, J. (1996). Should doctors guarantee results? or, whose disease is it, anyway? *Managed Care, 5*(12), 53–54.

Lee, V., Cohen, R., Edgar, L., Laizner, A. M., & Gagnon, A. J. (2006). Meaning-making and psychological adjustment to cancer: Development of an intervention and pilot results. *Oncology Nursing Forum, 33*(2), 291–302.

Levine, E. G. (2001). *Jewish perspectives on illness and healing.* New York: Rutledge.

Lo, B., Kates, L. W., Ruston, D., Arnold, R. M., Cohen, C., Puchalski, C. M., Pantilat, S. Z., Rabow, M. W., Schreiber, R. S., (2003). Responding to requests regarding prayer and religious ceremonies by patients near the end of life and their families. *Journal of Palliative Medicine, 6*(3), 409–415.

Lo, B., Quill, T., & Tulsky, J. (1999). Discussing palliative care with patients. *Annals of Internal Medicine, 130*(9), 744–749.

Lo, B., Ruston, D., Kates, L. W., Arnold, R. M., Cohen, C. B., Faber-Langendoen, K., Pantilat, S. Z., Puchalski, C. M., Quill, T. R., Rabow, M. W., Schreiber, S., Sulmasy, D. P., Tulsky, J. A. (2002). Discussing religious and spiritual issues at the end of life: A practical guide for physicians. *Journal of the American Medical Association, 287*(6), 749–754.

Lonergan, B. J. F. (1958). *Insight: A study of human understanding*. San Francisco: Harper and Row.

Lucas, A. M. (2001). Introduction to the discipline for pastoral care giving. In L. VandeCreek & A. M. Lucas (Eds.), *The discipline for pastoral care giving* (pp. 1–33). Binghamton, NY: Haworth Press, Inc.

Lucas, C. (1985). Out at the edge: Notes on a paradigm shift. *Journal of Counseling and Development, 64*(3), 165–172.

Lunn, J. (2004). Spiritual care in a multi-religious context. *Journal of Pain & Palliative Care Pharmacotherapy, 17*(3–4), 153–166.

Marcel, G. (1949). *Being and having*. (K. Farrer, Trans.). Glasgow, Scotland: The University Press.

Marie Curie Cancer Care. (n.d.). *Spiritual and religious care competencies for specialist palliative care*. London: Marie Curie Cancer Care. Retrieved March 31, 2009, from http://www.mariecurie.org.uk/forhealthcareprofessionals/spiritualandreligiouscare/index.htm

Markus, H. R., & Kitayama, S. (1991). Culture and the self: Implications for cognition, emotion, and motivation. *Psychological Review, 98*(2), 224–253.

Marler, P. L., & Hadaway, C. K. (2002). Being religious or being spiritual in America: A zero-sum proposition? *Journal for the Scientific Study of Religion, 41*(2), 289–300.

Maslow, A. H. (1962). *Towards a psychology of being*. Princeton, NJ: Van Nostrand.

Maugans, T. A. (1996). The SPIRITual history. *Archives of Family Medicine, 5*(1), 11–16.

Mauk, K. L., & Schmidt, N. A. (2004). *Spiritual care in nursing practice*. Philadelphia, PA: Lippincott Williams & Wilkins.

May, R. (1969). *Existential psychology*. New York: Random House.

McCall, J. B. (2004). *Bereavement counseling: Pastoral care for complicated grieving*. New York: Haworth Press.

McCauley, J., Tarpley, M. J., Haaz, S., & Bartlett, S. J. (2008). Daily spiritual experiences of older adults with and without arthritis and the relationship to health outcomes. *Arthritis and Rheumatism, 59*(1), 122–128

McCord, G., Gilchrist, V. J., Grossman, S. D., King, B. D., McCormick, K. E., Oprandi, A. M., Schrop, S. L., Selius, B. A., Smucker, W. D., Weldy,

D. L., Amorn, M., Carter, M. A., Deak, A. J., Hefzy, H., Srivastava, M. (2004). Discussing spirituality with patients: A rational and ethical approach. *Annals of Family Medicine, 2*(4), 356–361.

McDonald, R. (2006). *The spirituality of community life: When we come 'round right.* Binghamton, NY: Haworth Pastoral Press.

McEwen, B. S. (1998). Protective and damaging effects of stress mediators. *New England Journal of Medicine, 38*(3), 171–179.

McEwen, B. S., & Stellar, E.(1993). Stress and the individual: Mechanisms leading to disease. *Archives of Internal Medicine, 153*(18), 2093–2101.

McGrath, P. (2002). Creating a language for "spiritual pain" through research: A beginning. *Supportive Care in Cancer, 10*(8), 637–646.

McGrath, P. (2004). Positive outcomes for survivors of haematological malignancies from a spiritual perspective. *International Journal of Nursing Practice, 10*(6), 280–291.

Mckee, D. D., & Chappel, J. N. (1992). Spirituality and medical practice. *Journal of Family Practice, 35*(2), 201, 205–208.

McNeill, D. P., Morrison, D., & Nouwen, H. J. M. (2005). *Compassion: A reflection on the Christian life.* New York: Doubleday.

McNeill, J. A., Sherwood, G. D., Starck, P. L., & Thompson, C. J. (1998). Assessing clinical outcomes: Patient satisfaction with pain management. *Journal of Pain and Symptom Management, 16*(1), 29–40.

Meier, D. E., Back, A. L., & Morrison, R. S. (2001). The inner life of physicians and care of the seriously ill. *Journal of the American Medical Association, 286*(23), 3007–3014.

Miller, B. (2005). Spiritual journey during and after cancer treatment. *Gynecologic Oncology, 99*(3), Suppl 1, S129–S130.

Milliken, F. J., & Martins, L. L. (1996). Searching for common threads: Understanding the multiple effects of diversity in organizational groups. *The Academy of Management Review, 21*(2), 402–433.

Milstein, J. M. (2008). Introducing spirituality in medical care: Transition from hopelessness to wholeness. *Journal of the American Medical Association, 299*(20), 2440–2441.

Moore, T. (1996). *The education of the heart.* New York: HarperCollins Publishers.

Moss, B. (2005). *Religion and spirituality.* Lyme Regis, UK: Russell House Publishing.

Nagai-Jacobson, M. G., & Burkhardt, M. A. (1989). Spirituality: Cornerstone of holistic nursing practice. *Holistic Nursing Practice, 3*(3), 18–26.

NANDA International. (2007). *NANDA-I nursing diagnoses: Definitions and classification, 2007–2008.* Philadelphia: NANDA International.

National Association of Social Workers. (2008). Code of ethics. Retrieved

December 10, 2008, from http://www.socialworkers.org/pubs/code/ code.asp

National Comprehensive Cancer Network. (2008). NCCN clinical practice guidelines in oncology: Distress management. Retrieved March 31, 2009, from http://www.nccn.org/professionals/physician_gls/PDF/ distress.pdf

National Comprehensive Cancer Network (NCCN). (2009). *Palliative care.* Retrieved March 31, 2009, from http://www.nccn.org/professionals/ physician_gls/PDF/palliative.pdf

National Consensus Project (NCP) for Quality Palliative Care. (2004). National consensus project for quality palliative care: Clinical practice guidelines for quality palliative care, executive summary (Policy Document). *Journal of Palliative Medicine, 7*(5), 611–627.

National Consensus Project (NCP) for Quality Palliative Care Guidelines. (2009). Retrieved March 31, 2009, from www .nationalconsensusproject.org

National Interfaith Coalition on Aging (NICA). (1975). *Spiritual well-being.*

National Quality Forum (NQF). (2006). *A national framework and preferred practices for palliative and hospice care: A consensus report.* Washington DC: National Quality Forum. Retrieved August 28, 2008, from http://www.qualityforum.org/Publications/2006/12/A_ National_Framework_and_Preferred_Practices_for_Palliative_and_ Hospice_Care_Quality.aspx

Nelson-Becker, H. (2003). Practical philosophies: Interpretations of religion and spirituality by African-American and Jewish elders. *Journal of Religious Gerontology, 14*(2/3), 85–99.

Nelson-Becker, H. (2004). Spiritual, religious, nonspiritual, nonreligious narratives in marginalized older adults: A typology of coping styles. *Journal of Religion, Spirituality, and Aging, 17*(1/2), 21–38.

Nelson-Becker, H. (2006). Voices of resilience: Older adults in hospice care. *Journal of Social Work in End-of-Life & Palliative Care, 2*(3), 87–106.

Nelson-Becker, H. (2008). Integrating spirituality in practice: From inner journey to outer engagement. *Journal of Geriatric Care Management, 10*(2), 10–15.

Nelson-Becker, H., & Canda, E. R. (2008). Research on religion, spirituality, and aging: A social work perspective on the state of the art. *Journal of Religion, Spirituality, & Aging, 20*(3), 77.

Nelson-Becker, H., Nakashima, M., & Canda, E. R. (2006). Spirituality in professional helping interventions. In B. Berkman & S. D'Ambruoso (Eds.), *Handbook of social work in health and aging* (pp. 797–807). New York: Oxford University Press.

Netting, F. E., & Williams, F. (1996). Case manager-physician collaboration: Implications for professional identity, roles, and relationships. *Health & Social Work, 21*(3), 216–224.

Neuman, B. M. (1995). *The Neuman system model.* Stamford, CT: Appleton & Lange.

Nisbett, R. E., & Masuda, T. (2003). Culture and point of view. *Proceedings of the National Academy of Sciences of the United States of America, 100*(19), 11163–11170.

O'Brien, M. E. (1999). *Spirituality in nursing: Standing on holy ground.* Sudbury, MA: Jones and Bartlett.

O'Connor, A. P., & Wicker, C. A. (1995). Clinical commentary: Promoting meaning in the lives of cancer survivors. *Seminars in Oncology Nursing, 11*(1), 68–72.

O'Connor, P. (1988). The role of spiritual care in hospice: Are we meeting patients' needs? *American Journal of Hospice Care, 5*(4), 31–37.

O'Donnell, E. (2007). *Spirituality and human development: Course for spirituality and health online graduate certificate program.* Washington, DC: George Washington University.

Otis-Green, S. (2006). The transitions program: Existential care in action. *Journal of Cancer Education, 21*(1), 23–25.

Otis-Green, S. (2007). Guest editorial. *American Academy of Pain Management: The Pain Practitioner, 17*(2), 7.

Otis-Green, S., Ferrell, B., Spolum, M., Mullan, P., Baird, P., & Grant, M. (2009). An overview of the ACE project—Advocating for clinical excellence: Transdisciplinary palliative care education. *Journal of Cancer Education, 24*(2), 120–126.

Otis-Green, S., Sherman, R., Perez, M., & Baird, R. P. (2002). An integrated psychosocial-spiritual model for cancer pain management. *Cancer Practice, 10*(Suppl 1), S58–65.

Padmasambhava. (2005). *The Tibetan book of the dead.* London: Penguin Books.

Pannuti, F., & Tanneberger, S. (1993). Dying with dignity: Illusion, hope or human right? *World Health Forum, 14*(2), 172–173.

Pargament, K. (1997). *The psychology of religion and coping: Theory, research, practice.* New York: Guilford Publications.

Pargament, K. I., Koenig, H. G., Tarakeshwar, N., & Hahn, J. (2001). Religious struggle as a predictor of mortality among medically ill elderly patients: A two-year longitudinal study. *Archives of Internal Medicine, 161*(15), 1881–1885.

Pargament, K. I., Koenig, H. G., Tarakeshwar, N., & Hahn, J. (2004). Religious coping methods as predictors of psychological, physical and spiritual outcomes among medically ill elderly patients: A two-year longitudinal study. *Journal of Health Psychology, 9*(6), 713–730.

Pargament, K. I., Smith, B. W., Koenig, H. G., & Perez, L. (1998). Patterns of negative and religious coping with major life stressors. *Journal for the Scientific Study of Religion* 37(4), 710–724.

Park, C. L., & Folkman, S. (1997). Meaning in the context of stress and coping. *Review of General Psychology, 1*(2), 115–144.

Park, J. (2007). *Opening to grace: Transcending our spiritual malaise.* Minneapolis: Existential Books.

Payne, M. (2000). *Teamwork in multiprofessional care.* Chicago: Lyceum Books.

Penson, R. T., Dignan, F. L., Canellos, G. P., Picard, C. L., & Lynch, T. J., Jr. (2000). Burnout: Caring for the caregivers. *Oncologist, 5*(5), 425–434.

Phelps, A. C., Maciejewski, P. K., Nilsson, M., Balboni, T. A., Wright, A. A., Paulk, M. E., Trice, E., Schrag, D., Peteet, J., Block, S. D., Prigerson, H. G. (2009). Religious coping and use of intensive life-prolonging care near death in patients with advanced cancer. *JAMA: The Journal of the American Medical Association, 301*(11), 1140–1147.

Powell, L. H., Shahabi, L., & Thoresen, C. E. (2003). Religion and spirituality: Linkages to physical health. *American Psychologist, 58*(1), 36–52.

Prince-Paul, M. (2008). Understanding the meaning of social well-being at the end of life. *ONF, 35*(3), 365–371.

Pruyser, P. W. (1976). *The minister as diagnostician.* Philadelphia: Westminster Press.

Puchalski, C. (2002a). Forgiveness: spiritual and medical implications. *The Yale Journal for Humanities in Medicine.* Retrieved March 31, 2009, from http://yjhm.yale.edu/archives/spirit2003/forgiveness/cpuchalski.htm

Puchalski, C. (2002b). Spirituality. In A. Berger, R. Portenoy, & D. Weissman (Eds.), *Principles and practice of palliative care and supportive oncology* (2nd ed., pp. 799–812). Philadelphia: Lippincott Williams & Wilkins.

Puchalski, C. (2004). Spirituality in health: The role of spirituality in critical care. *Critical Care Clinics, 20*(3), 487–504.

Puchalski, C. (2006a). Spiritual assessment in clinical practice. *Psychiatric Annals, 36*(3), 150.

Puchalski, C. (2006b). Spirituality and medicine: Curricula in medical education. *Journal of Cancer Education, 21*(1), 14–18.

Puchalski, C. (2006c). *A time for listening and caring: Spirituality and the care of the chronically ill and dying.* New York: Oxford University Press.

Puchalski, C. (2007). Spirituality and the care of patients at the end-of-life: An essential component of care. *Omega: Journal of Death and Dying, 56*(1), 33–46.

Puchalski, C. (2008). Honoring the sacred in medicine: Spirituality as an essential element of patient-centered care. *Journal of Medicine and the Person, 6*(3), 113–117.

Puchalski, C. & Blatt, J. (2000). *The practice of medicine curriculum for medical students.* Washington, DC: The George Washington University School of Medicine.

Puchalski, C., Dorff, R. E., & Hendi, I. Y. (2004). Spirituality, religion, and healing in palliative care. *Clinics in Geriatric Medicine, 20*(4), 689–714.

Puchalski, C. M., Ferrell, B., Virani, R., Otis-Green, S., Baird, P., & Bull, J. (2009). Improving the quality of spiritual care as a dimension of palliative care: Consensus conference report. *Journal of Palliative Medicine, 12*(10), 885–903.

Puchalski, C., Kilpatrick, S. D., McCullough, M. E., & Larson, D. B. (2003). A systematic review of spiritual and religious variables in *Palliative Medicine, American Journal of Hospice and Palliative Care, Hospice Journal, Journal of Palliative Care,* and *Journal of Pain and Symptom Management. Palliative & Supportive Care, 1*(1), 7–13.

Puchalski, C., & Larson, D. B. (1998). Developing curricula in spirituality and medicine. *Academic Medicine, 73*(9), 970–974.

Puchalski, C., & Lunsford, B. (2008). *White paper on spirituality and compassion.* Kalamazoo, MI: Fetzer Institute.

Puchalski, C., Lunsford, B., Harris, M. H., & Miller, R. T. (2006). Interdisciplinary spiritual care for seriously ill and dying patients: A collaborative model. *Cancer Journal, 12*(5), 398–416.

Puchalski, C., & McSkimming, S. (2006). Creating healing environments. *Health Progress, 87*(3), 30–35.

Puchalski, C., & O'Donnell, E. (2005). Religious and spiritual beliefs in end of life care: How major religions view death and dying. *Techniques in Regional Anesthesia and Pain Management, 9*(3), 114–121.

Puchalski, C., & Romer, A. L. (2000). Taking a spiritual history allows clinicians to understand patients more fully. *Journal of Palliative Medicine, 3*(1), 129–137.

Ramsey, P. (1970). *The patient as person: Explorations in medical ethics.* New Haven, CT: Yale University Press.

Rancour, P. (2008). Using archetypes and transitions theory to help move from active treatment to survivorship. *Clinical Journal of Oncology Nursing, 12*(6), 935–940.

Reed, P. G. (1987). Spirituality and well-being in terminally ill hospitalized adults. *Research in Nursing & Health, 10*(5), 335–344.

Reed, P. G. (1992). An emerging paradigm for the investigation of spirituality in nursing. *Research in Nursing & Health, 15*(5), 349–357

Registered Nurse Central Online. (2007). *Spiritual distress.* Retrieved

August 21, 2009, from http://www.rncentral.com/nursing-library/careplans/sd

Richards, P. S., & Bergin, A. E. (2002). *A spiritual strategy for counseling and psychotherapy*. Washington, DC: American Psychological Association.

Ritual. (2008). In *Merriam-Webster online*. Retrieved February 10, 2009, from http://www.merriam-webster.com/

Roberts, J. A., Brown, D., Elkins, T., & Larson, D. B. (1997). Factors influencing views of patients with gynecologic cancer about end-of-life decisions. *American Journal of Obstetrics & Gynecology, 176*(1, Part 1), 166–172.

Rodgers, B. L., & Knafl, K. A. (1993). *Concept development in nursing*. London: Saunders.

Sabo, B. M. (2006). Compassion fatigue and nursing work: Can we accurately capture the consequences of caring work? *International Journal of Nursing Practice, 12*(3), 136–142.

Sachedina, A. (2005). End-of-life: The Islamic view. *The Lancet, 366*(9487), 774–779.

Sanghavi, D. M. (2006). What makes for a compassionate patient-caregiver relationship? *Joint Commission Journal on Quality & Patient Safety, 32*(5), 283–292.

Sawatzky, R., & Pesut, B. (2005). Attributes of spiritual care in nursing practice. *Journal of Holistic Nursing, 23*(1), 19–33.

Schneider, R. H., Alexander, C. N., Staggers, F., Rainforth, M., Salerno, J. W., Hartz, A., ... Nidich, S. I. (2005). Long-term effects of stress reduction on mortality in persons > or = 55 years of age with systemic hypertension. *American Journal of Cardiology, 95*(9), 1060–1064.

Schweitzer, A. (1931). *The primeval forest*. New York: Macmillan Company.

Seeman, T. E., Aubin, L. F., & Seema, M. (2003). Religiosity/spirituality and health: A critical review of the evidence for biological pathways. *American Psychologist, 58*(1), 53–63.

Senesh, H. (2004). *Hannah Senesh: Her life and diary*. Woodstock, VT: Jewish Lights Publishing.

Shafranske, E. P. (1996). *Religion and the clinical practice of psychology*. Washington, DC: American Psychological Association.

Sherman, A. C., Simonton, S., Latif, U., Spohn, R., & Tricot, G. (2005). Religious struggle and religious comfort in response to illness: Health outcomes among stem cell transplant patients. *Journal of Behavioral Medicine, 28*(4), 359–367.

Silvestri, G. A., Knittig, S., Zoller, J. S., & Nietert, P. J. (2003). Importance of faith on medical decisions regarding cancer care. *Journal of Clinical Oncology, 21*(7), 1379–1382.

Sivananda, S. S. (2000). *Bhagavad Gita*. Himalayas, India: The Divine Life Society.

Skalla, K., & McCoy, J. (2006). Spiritual assessment of patients with cancer: The moral authority, vocation, aesthetic, social, and transcendent model. *Oncology Nursing Forum, 33*(4), 745–751.

Sloan, R. P., Bagiella, E., VandeCreek, L., Hover, M., Casalone, C., Jinpu Hirsch, T., Hasan, Y., Kreger, R., Poulos, P. (2000). Should physicians prescribe religious activity? *New England Journal of Medicine, 342*(25), 1913–1916.

Smith, A. R. (2006). Using the synergy model to provide spiritual nursing care in critical care settings. *Critical Care Nurse, 26*(4), 41–47.

Smith, W. J. (2005). Dame Cecily Saunders: The mother of modern hospice care passes on. *The Weekly Standard*. Retrieved March 31, 2009, from http://www.weeklystandard.com/Content/Public/Articles/000/000/005/846ozowf.asp

Snyder, C. R., Irving, L. M., & Anderson, J. R. (1991). Hope and health: Measuring the will and the ways. In C. R. Snyder & D. R. Forsyth (Eds.), *Handbook of social and clinical psychology: The health perspective* (pp. 285–307). Elmsford, NY: Pergamon Press.

Social Connectedness. (2009). In *The free dictionary online*. Retrieved August 21, 2009, from http://encyclopedia.thefreedictionary.com/Social+connectedness

Spilka, B., Shaver, P., & Kirkpatrick, L. A. (1985). A general attribution theory for the psychology of religion. *Journal for the Scientific Study of Religion, 24*(1), 1–20.

Spiritual Care Collaborative—Standards. (2007). Available from http://www.spiritualcarecollaborative.org/standards.asp

Steel, J., Gamblin, C., & Carr, B. (2008). Measuring post-traumatic growth in people diagnosed with hepatobiliary cancer: Directions for future research. *Oncology Nursing Forum, 35*(4), 643–650.

Stewart, M.A. (1995). Effective physician-patient communication and health outcomes: A review. *CMAJ Canadian Medical Association Journal, 152*(9), 1423–1433.

Strada, E. A. (2008). Preserving life at the end of life: Shifting the temporal dimension of hope. *Palliative & Supportive Care, 6*(2), 187–188.

Strada, E. A., & Sourkes, B. (2009). Principles of psychotherapy. In J. Holland (Ed.), *Psycho-oncology* (2nd ed.). New York: Oxford.

Sulmasy, D. P. (1999). Is medicine a spiritual practice? *Academic Medicine, 74*(9), 1002–1005.

Sulmasy, D. P. (2000). Healing the dying: Spiritual issues in the care of the dying patient. In J. Kissel & D. C. Thomasma (Eds.), *The health professional as friend and healer* (pp. 188–197). Washington, DC: Georgetown University Press.

Sulmasy, D. P. (2001). At wit's end: Dignity, forgiveness, and the care of the dying. *Journal of General Internal Medicine, 16*(5), 335–338.

Sulmasy, D. P. (2002). A biopsychosocial-spiritual model for the care of patients at the end of life. *Gerontologist, 42*(3), 24–33.

Sulmasy, D. P. (2006). *The rebirth of the clinic: An introduction to spirituality in healthcare.* Washington, DC: Georgetown University Press.

Sulmasy, D. P., Geller, G., Levine, D. M., & Faden, R. (1992). The quality of mercy: Caring for patients with do not resuscitate orders. *Journal of the American Medical Association, 267*(5), 682–686.

Sumner, C. H. (1998). Recognizing and responding to spiritual distress. *The American Journal of Nursing, 98*(1), 26–30.

Swift, C., Calcutawalla, S., & Elliot, R. (2007). Nursing attitudes towards recording of religious and spiritual data. *British Journal of Nursing, 16*(20), 1279–1282.

Tatsumura, Y., Maskarinec, G., Shumay, D. M., & Kakai, H. (2003). Religious and spiritual resources, CAM, and conventional treatment in the lives of cancer patients. *Alternative Therapies in Health and Medicine, 9*(3), 64–71.

Taylor, E. J. (2001). *Spiritual care: Nursing theory, research, and practice.* Saddle River, NJ: Prentice-Hall.

Taylor, E. J. (2003). Spiritual needs of patients with cancer and family caregivers. *Cancer Nursing, 26*(4), 260–266.

Tedeschi, R. G., & Calhoun, L. G. (1996). The posttraumatic growth inventory: Measuring the positive legacy of trauma. *Journal of Traumatic Stress, 9*(3), 455–471.

Teilhard de Chardin, P. (1960). *The devine milieu.* New York: Harper.

Tillich, P. (1963). The philosophy of social work. *Pastoral Psychology, 14*(9), 27–30.

Tinoco, L. (2006). *Providing culturally and linguistically competent health care.* Oakbrook Terrace, IL: Joint Commission Resources.

Tippett, K. (2007). *Speaking of faith.* New York: Penguin Books.

Tsevat, J., Sherman, S. N., McElwee, J. A., Mandell, K. L., Simbartl, L. A., Sonnenberg, F. A., Fowler, F. J. (1999). The will to live among HIV-infected patients. *Annals of Internal Medicine, 131*(3), 194–198.

Twaddle, M. L., Maxwell, T. L., Cassel, J. B., Liao, S., Coyne, P. J., Usher, B. M., Amin, A., Cuny, J. (2007). Palliative care benchmarks from academic medical centers. *Journal of Palliative Medicine, 10*(1), 86–98.

Underwood, L.G. (2005). Interviews with Trappist monks as a contribution to research methodology in the investigation of compassionate love. *Journal for the Theory of Social Behaviour, 35*(3), 285–302.

Unruh, A. M., Versnel, J., & Kerr, N. (2002). Spirituality unplugged: A review of commonalities and contentions, and a resolution. *Canadian Journal of Occupational Therapy—Revue Canadienne d Ergotherapie, 69*(1), 5–19.

Vachon, M. (2008). Meaning, spirituality, and wellness in cancer survivors. *Seminars in Oncology Nursing, 24*(3), 218–225.

Van der Hart, O. (1988). *Coping with loss: The therapeutic use of leave-taking rituals.* New York: Irvington.

VandeCreek, L., & Burton, L. (Eds.). (2001). Professional chaplaincy: Its role and importance in healthcare. Retrieved February 10, 2009, from http://www.healthcarechaplaincy.org/userimages/professional-chaplaincy-its-role-and-importance-in-healthcare.pdf

Vanistendael, S. (2007). Resilience and spirituality. In B. Monroe & D. Oliviere (Eds.), *Resilience in palliative care: Achievement in adversity* (pp. 115–136). Oxford: Oxford University Press.

Wald, F. S. (1998). The emergence of hospice care in the United States. In H. Spiro, M. G. Curnen, & L. P. Wandel (Eds.), *Facing death: Where culture, religion, and medicine meet.* (pp. 81–89). New Haven, CT: Yale University Press.

Waldfogel, S., & Wolpe, P. R. (1993). Using awareness of religious factors to enhance interventions in consultation-liaison psychiatry. *Hospital Community Psychiatry 44*(5), 473–477.

Watson, J. (1919). *Psychology from the standpoint of a behaviorist.* Philadelphia: Lippincott.

Watson, J. B. (1999). Becoming aware: Knowing yourself to care for others. *Home Healthcare Nurse, 17*(5), 317–322.

Weisman, A. D. (1972). *On dying and denying: A psychiatric study of terminality.* New York: Behavioral Publications.

Weissman, D. E., Ambuel, B., Von Gunten, C. F., Block, S., Warm, E., Hallenbeck, J., Milch, R., Brasel, K., Mullan, P. B. (2007). Outcomes from a national multispecialty palliative care curriculum development project. *Journal of Palliative Medicine, 10*(2), 408–419.

Weissman, D. E., Mullan, P., Ambuel, B., von Gunten, C. F., Hallenbeck, J., & Warm, E. (2001). End-of-life graduate education curriculum project: Project abstracts/progress reports—Year 2. *Journal of Palliative Medicine, 4*(4), 525–547.

White, K. L., Williams, T. F., & Greenberg, B. G. (1996). The ecology of medical care. *Bulletin of the New York Academy of Medicine, 73*(1), 187–205.

Wong, P. T. P., & Fry, P. S. (1998). *The human quest for meaning: A handbook of psychological research and clinical applications.* Mahwah, NJ: Lawrence Erlbaum Associates.

World Health Organization. (2007). *Cancer control: Knowledge into action: WHO guide for effective programmes; module 5*. Retrieved March 31, 2009, from http://www.who.int/cancer/media/FINAL-PalliativeCareModule.pdf

Worthington, E. L. (2001). *Five steps to forgiveness: The art and science of forgiving*. New York: Crown Publishers.

Wright, L. M. (2005). *Spirituality, suffering, and illness: Ideas for healing*. Philadelphia: F. A. Davis Co.

Yalom, I. D. (1980). *Existential psychotherapy*. New York: Basic Books.

Yang, K. A. (1995). *Taoism and health*. Heilungjiang: Xinhua Books.

Yates, J. W., Chalmer, B. J., & St. James, P. (1981). Religion in patients with advanced cancer. *Medical and Pediatric Oncology, 9*(2), 121–128.

Yi, M. S., Mrus, J. M., Mueller, C. V., Luckhaupt, S. E., Peterman, A. H., Puchalski, C. M., Tsevat, J. (2007). Self-rated health of primary care house officers and its relationship to psychological and spiritual well-being. *BMC Medical Education, 7*(9).

Zwingmann, C., Wirtz, M., Muller, C., Korber, J., & Murken, S. (2006). Positive and negative religious coping in German breast cancer patients. *Journal of Behavioral Medicine, 29*(6), 533–547.

Index

death *(cont.)*
  rituals of, 26
  spiritual care at time of, 61–62
  spiritual care of family after, 61
  spiritual preparation for, 26
demoralization syndrome
  approaches to, 24–25, 113
  definition of, 24
  as expression of existential
    distress, 113
denial, 50–51
depression
  in primary care physician
    residents, 175
  spirituality of physician residents
    influencing, 175
  therapeutic process and, 75
Descartes, Rene, 12
diagnosis coding, 125–26
dignity model of spiritual care
  categories of, 56
  for terminally ill patients, 55
Dignity-Conserving Practices Model,
  112–13
Discipline for Pastoral Care Giving
  (Lucas), 95
disease, 104
distancing, 43
  appropriate boundaries *vs.*, 42–43
  by clinicians, 42
divergent beliefs, 115
do not resuscitate orders, 91
documentation of patients' spiritual
  information
    in biopsychosocial-spiritual model
      of care, 137
    good, 135–36
    overall care through, 136
    time needed for, 135, 137
documentation of spiritual care
  biopsychosocial-spiritual care
    plan and, 133
  privacy in, 133, 135
  purpose of, 133, 135
Duke Institute on Care at the End of
  Life, 161
dying
  distanced from family and faith,
    29
  hospital's focus of care and, 29
  importance in, 30
  patient's spiritual goals when, 130

quality of life and, 29
religious/spiritual struggle
  triggered by, 77–78
spiritual care of, 141
spiritual issues faced by, 76
spirituality and, 3–4, 31–32
translocation of care for, 29

ecologic model of patient care, 103
end of life
  ACP consensus panel on, 57
  biopsychosocial-spiritual model of
    care at, 108
  care by psychologists at, 39
  community religious leaders role
    at, 160–61
  core values of, 35
  courses in care at, 155–56,
    156–57
  Duke Institute on Care at, 161
  existential questions at, 79
  health care system at, 155
  meaning and purpose of life at,
    74
  Nursing Education Consortium
    and, 157
  nursing practice at, 34–35
  physician assistants' care at, 39
  psychologists and, 161–62
  ritual at, 122
  spiritual care at, 79–80
  spiritual growth at, 82
  statistics of courses on care at,
    155–56
  team care at, 140–42
End-of-Life Nursing Education
  Consortium, 157
Engel, George, 103
*Essentials of Baccalaureate Education
  for Professional Nursing Practice*,
  157
ethical guidelines. *See also* code of
  ethics
    clinician/patient power imbalance
      and, 40
    for clinicians, 40
    intimacy of spirituality and, 40
    proselytizing and, 44–45
    for psychologists, 38
    spiritual care needs of patients
      and, 40
    spiritual practices and, 123